ACHIEVE LEAN
PLAN FOR HEALTHY EATING
By Anne Johns

Please consult with your physician prior to starting this Plan.

PREFACE

I have worked with many clients of all ages, sizes and fitness levels helping them find their paths to a lifetime of health, wellness and fitness. I have observed a common denominator for those individuals who have tried and tried again to lose fat and become leaner and stronger. Their inability to succeed is not due to lack of motivation or trying all manner of diets. The greatest hurdle for many is their unhealthy relationship with food: emotional eating; stress eating; celebratory eating.

This eight-week Plan is designed to reorient your relationship with food. The process is simple and the change in perspective happens naturally, with very little effort. The end result is health, wellness, strength, functionality and a lean physique.

I dedicate this book to each of you who feel that you will never be able to succeed. You can and you will.

Please visit my website if you would like to purchase online coaching to supplement this book.

www.achievelean.net

TABLE OF CONTENTS

INTRODUCTION

THE PLAN

The Achieve Lean Plan for Healthy Eating will simplify your relationship with food and possibly your life. Too often, we complicate our lives with food. We skip breakfast, which leads to binge eating and feelings of guilt and self-punishment. We postpone eating during our busy days until we are weak with hunger, headache, and irritability; then we grab whatever is available and engage in uncontrolled eating.

We treat food as a friend or enemy depending on the moment. If we are feeling up, we eat – if we are feeling down, we eat. We pamper ourselves with treats of the worse kind. No sooner do we befriend food – enjoying it with reckless abandon – we despise it because we overindulged. Food is a powerful companion in our lives! More powerful than you may realize; it is ultimately the difference between sickness and wellness.

Achieve Lean will help you change your relationship with food. Healthy food is fuel for the brain and body. It makes us strong, vibrant, happy, sexy, and well. Although we've convinced ourselves otherwise, healthy food is truly tasty and satisfying.

Achieve Lean is not a plan of self-deprivation. It is a plan that teaches systematic eating and awareness of each and every food choice we make. The goal of Achieve Lean is to create health and wellness, and the result is a leaner, stronger body. The fewer unhealthy foods you choose to eat, the healthier and leaner you will become.

Achieve Lean establishes eating awareness – the first step in creating change. Your work is to write down every food item at the moment it is consumed. This is work you cannot avoid. Take your journal everywhere – do not promise yourself that you will remember and make record later. You won't remember, and you won't be in the moment with your eating.

Follow the schedule of eating. You may not be hungry when the schedule requires you to eat. Eat anyway. You are training new habits. In time, your body will adjust, and you will find that you become hungry at the appropriate times.

Once you have established eating awareness and a schedule of eating, we begin to adjust the quality of food choices. The first macronutrient that we address is protein. Achieve Lean focuses on animal proteins as they are the best for muscle growth and exercise support. You cannot lose fat without gaining muscle. Many individuals progressively lose muscle due to lack of protein in the daily diet, poor eating habits and improper exercise. Don't worry that you might get bulky with more protein. You won't.

The body needs water not only for protein assimilation, but for overall wellness. Your body does not run well if you do not drink between ½ to a full gallon of water daily. Before each meal, you will consume 16 ounces of water guaranteeing that you reach your daily requirement by the final meal. The time you spend drinking your water and reciting your intention will calm you down and will fill you up before sitting down to your meal. You will therefore have a more satisfying meal experience and will not crave more food after the meal. If you don't like water, learn to – it's required.

Achieve Lean helps you create a healthy digestive system. A clogged system is an unhealthy system and cannot support lean gains. We introduce vegetables, non-digestible fibers and fish oil capsules – all supporting a clean digestive system. You will be amazed at how healthy you feel each morning if your system is running free and clear! Teach yourself to like vegetables – you absolutely need them. No vegetable makes you fat, and all of them contribute greatly to a healthy, lean body.

Once we establish the eating schedule and the foods we need to become lean and healthy, we begin to slowly subtract the foods that are making us fat. At this point in the Plan, you will be ready to do that. You will be experiencing positive changes in your body and in your health, and you will be motivated to rid your diet of most or all of the junk. You'll be ready to commit to getting and staying lean!

Achieve Lean is an eight-week plan that teaches you to establish a systematic pattern of eating and a healthy relationship with food. However, should you need more time, take it. You can and should repeat any week if you feel the need. Progress should be as slow as necessary to support continuing success. The changes that you make are intended to be life long and the effort worthwhile. Take your time and enjoy the process.

GENTLE DISCIPLINE

Healthy eating is an ongoing process comprised of peaks and valleys. Your current weight and body composition, age, activity level, exercise frequency and intensity, and whether you have any injuries are all factors that contribute to how quickly and easily you can obtain a state of wellness and the resulting lean physique. Nurture yourself; give yourself plenty of time to succeed. Recognize that your relationship with food may get in the way of following the plan. Don't punish yourself if you fall off the plan; simply get back on it immediately. Give yourself credit for doing the best you can. Continue trying and don't give up.

Achieve Lean gets you started on the process of creating lifelong, healthy eating. The plan has few parameters, but they are strict and must be adhered to in order to succeed. Once you consistently follow the parameters – daily consumption of water, protein, vegetables, fiber and fish oil combined with systematic eating – you have freedom to experiment with other foods to see what works for you.

You cannot achieve a healthy, lean state without discipline. But discipline is not denial nor is it deprivation. Be patient, and be kind; gently teach yourself the discipline needed to follow this Plan.

THE INTENTIONS, MEDITATION AND CONSCIOUS EATING

Achieve Lean teaches awareness. Meditation is a large part of creating awareness. Meditation is a universal healer and is an integral part of a lifetime of wellness.

Achieve Lean begins your meditation practice with weekly intentions. Recite each intention both aloud and silently. You can recite aloud in the shower or in your car – this way you can associate the recitations with a daily activity. Recite the intention silently as you are drinking your water prior to each meal. This will set the stage for a calmer, more conscious eating experience, devoid of cravings. As often as possible, sit down quietly and simply eat. Focus on your food and the eating experience. Remove the clutter – no television, no computer, no distractions!

I encourage you to take your meditation a step farther and carve out a few minutes every single day to sit quietly. Sit or lie down comfortably and breathe in and out as slowly and fully as you can. You will find in time, your breath will travel deeper into the lungs and will become slower. As you breathe in, silently recite the weekly intention. As you breathe out, silently say the number of the breath. Practice this for 9-36 breaths.

Practicing meditation and the intentions will naturally cause your behavior to change. Your mind quiets and you are less prone to make hasty, reactive responses. You become more objective and more present. Anxiety decreases and food cravings are diminished.

REDEFINING YOUR RELATIONSHIP WITH FOOD

We are a culture of emotional eaters. As children, we were given treats when we felt sad to help us feel better. We were given treats to celebrate our accomplishments. The dinner table was often a battleground. You could not receive your coveted dessert if you first did not consume all that was on your plate, including the despised vegetables. We were taught to hate the sustenance and to love the junk.

For many of us, this emotional relationship with food is powerful and will be the greatest hurdle to overcome. Mastering a healthy relationship takes a tremendous amount of work. Achieve Lean simplifies the process by allowing you to focus on awareness of eating habits and creating systematic behaviors. Positive action and thought helps to create long-term behavioral changes.

EAT SYSTEMATICALLY

Our days are busy and we often eat on the run or around social events. It may seem that your current lifestyle may not be compatible with systematic eating. It can be – you just have to teach yourself new habits. Always carry water and protein powder. When it is time to eat and you find yourself unable to sit down to a meal, drink your protein. These days it is quite acceptable to have a water bottle in your hand – you can use an opaque bottle so no one will know you are consuming protein.

If you have a planned social event that includes eating, do not postpone your meal. Eat a small meal prior to leaving for the event or drink some protein. This habit will keep you on schedule and will keep you from over consuming both food and drink during the event.

EAT AS FRESH AS POSSIBLE

Fresh, clean foods are those that move directly from the earth to your table. Locate meats, dairy items, fruits and vegetables that are sold by the farmers who raise the animals and grow the crops. Learn whether the farmer uses pesticides and if possible, find and purchase organic.

I live on Maryland's Eastern Shore, and we are very lucky to have fish that is caught from the Chesapeake Bay and sold locally. We have plenty of farm land and farmers who are raising healthy meats and produce. Even if you don't live in a rural area, you can find a way to obtain these foods online.

Many of us have plenty of packaged food in our kitchens. These foods are processed and do not contribute to lean gains. It can be argued that some of these foods, like whole grains provide necessary nutrients in the diet. Many of you will desire to keep some of these healthier processed foods in your daily eating. Achieve Lean allows for this choice.

If you want to keep whole grain breads in your diet, either make your own or choose products that are close to homemade. The ingredient list will be short and there will be no artificial additives and preservatives.

CHOOSE YOUR TEAM

Support is critical for success. If you are coaching with me, I represent your primary mode of support. I will be available to you daily by text or email to answer any questions and to motivate you towards success every day, every meal. I will also provide you with proper exercise programming (if applicable) and the motivation to complete each session. Proper exercise is instrumental to your success.

Find as many individuals who will understand, respect and support your efforts. If your loved ones are not ready to participate in Achieve Lean, find strategies that will help you to succeed. Creating separate cupboards for your foods and theirs will keep the unhealthy foods out of your line of sight. Take a walk or move to another room if your family member is having a treat that weakens your resolve. Often, when your family members see the improvements in you, they will begin to follow your lead and will join your efforts.

GET OFF THE SCALE!

Are you addicted to your scale? Do you weigh yourself every day and then admonish yourself if you gained a pound? Too often, the scale is the focal point that feeds our frustrations.

Individuals who focus on scale weight will likely lose precious muscle tissue and become skinny fat. The frame may get smaller, but the body composition remains relatively high. This is not healthy!

We record scale weight at the beginning and end of the eight weeks. We track lean gains weekly using three measurements: waist, abdomen and hip. These measurements are the best indicators of fat loss and keep you on the right track.

ACHIEVE LEAN IS YOUR REALITY

Any change is difficult, but the effort that you put into this Plan will pay off abundantly. As with creating any change, Achieve Lean will take some effort. This Plan is based on long-term behavior change, not short-term deprivation and quick results.

If you use all the resources available to you with Achieve Lean and take it one step at a time, you will find that you, too, can Achieve Lean!

WEEK ONE: Achieve a healthy schedule of eating

The first step in achieving a healthy relationship with food is learning to treat it as the sustenance that it is. This attitude requires that you learn to eat when necessary for the body's health, not when you feel like it or when you are famished.

Systematic eating is very important for health and lean gains. The Plan establishes a habit of eating small meals every two to three hours. This method of eating diminishes cravings, naturally keeps portion sizes down and calms out-of-control eating.

Consume 16 ounces of water prior to each meal. Although you may consume other liquids throughout your day, and all non-alcoholic liquids are good except for sodas – which have absolutely no place in a healthy diet – we count only the water. If you hit the baseline water consumption of 16 ounces five meals daily, you will be getting the recommended amount of half gallon of water daily. Consuming liquids beyond that is beneficial but not required and therefore is not included in the Plan.

Recite the weekly intention. Positive affirmations are the foundation for creating positive action and behavior. As you drink your water, silently repeat the intention 3 times. Recite the intention 5 times in the mornings and evenings. Do this in the shower, in your car, while you are preparing a meal. Associate the intention with an established activity so that it becomes a habit. If you do this with consistency and meaning, by the end of the week, you will feel calmer and more secure in your readiness to change your eating habits.

Creating awareness of your eating may be the most difficult step. Write down every single food item consumed when it is consumed. This is the only way to increase your awareness, which is an important step in changing food choices. Approach this task as objectively as possible – you are simply observing what you eat, not making judgments about it.

At the end of the week, take a close look at your food choices and notice if you had a trend towards change by the week's end. Do nothing more than observe and learn from what you recorded. Make no judgments or declarations for doing things differently or better. Trust that the knowledge of what you ate for the week is enough to help enact change.

To sum up, by the end of Week One, you will have established:
- Systematic eating including consuming within one hour of awakening and consuming every 2-3 hours thereafter
- Consuming 16 ounces of water prior to each meal
- Reciting and benefitting from the intentions, 5 times each in morning and night and 3 times prior to eating
- Greater awareness of food choices at each meal

WEEK ONE: Achieve a healthy schedule of eating

DAY ONE: _____

WEEK ONE INTENTION (Repeat aloud 5 times in the morning and 5 times at night. Repeat silently 3 times prior to each meal):
I CREATE HEALTHY HABITS FOR MYSELF (AND MY FAMILY)

Abdomen msmt: _____   **Waist msmt:** _____   **Hip msmt:** _____

Meal #1 (within one hour of awakening) Time: _____   Water = 16 oz.
(must be completely consumed prior to eating)
Write down all foods consumed:

_____

_____

_____

_____

Meal #2 (3 hours later) Time: _____
Water = 16 oz. (must be completely consumed prior to eating)
Write down all foods consumed:

_____

_____

_____

_____

Meal #3 (3 hours later) Time: _____
Water = 16 oz. (must be completely consumed prior to eating)
Write down all foods consumed:

_____

_____

_____

_____

Meal #4 (3 hours later) Time: _____
Water = 16 oz. (must be completely consumed prior to eating)
Write down all foods consumed:

_____

_____

_____

_____

_____

Meal #5 (3 hours later) Time: _____
Water = 16 oz. (must be completely consumed prior to eating)
Write down all foods consumed:

_____

_____

_____

_____

_____

WEEK ONE: Achieve a healthy schedule of eating

DAY TWO: _____

WEEK ONE INTENTION (Repeat aloud 5 times in the morning and 5 times at night. Repeat silently 3 times prior to each meal):

I CREATE HEALTHY HABITS FOR MYSELF (AND MY FAMILY)

Meal #1 (within one hour of awakening) Time: _____
Water = 16 oz. (must be completely consumed prior to eating)
Write down all foods consumed:

_____

_____

_____

_____

Meal #2 (3 hours later) Time: _____
Water = 16 oz. (must be completely consumed prior to eating)
Write down all foods consumed:

_____

_____

_____

_____

Meal #3 (3 hours later) Time: _____
Water = 16 oz. (must be completely consumed prior to eating)
Write down all foods consumed:

_____

_____

_____

_____

Meal #4 (3 hours later) Time: _____
Water = 16 oz. (must be completely consumed prior to eating)
Write down all foods consumed:

_____

_____

_____

_____

_____

Meal #5 (3 hours later) Time: _____
Water = 16 oz. (must be completely consumed prior to eating)
Write down all foods consumed:

_____

_____

_____

_____

_____

WEEK ONE: Achieve a healthy schedule of eating

DAY THREE: _____

WEEK ONE INTENTION (Repeat aloud 5 times in the morning and 5 times at night. Repeat silently 3 times prior to each meal):

I CREATE HEALTHY HABITS FOR MYSELF (AND MY FAMILY)

Meal #1 (within one hour of awakening) Time: _____
Water = 16 oz. (must be completely consumed prior to eating)
Write down all foods consumed:

_____

_____

_____

_____

Meal #2 (3 hours later) Time: _____
Water = 16 oz. (must be completely consumed prior to eating)
Write down all foods consumed:

_____

_____

_____

_____

Meal #3 (3 hours later) Time: _____
Water = 16 oz. (must be completely consumed prior to eating)
Write down all foods consumed:

_____

_____

_____

_____

Meal #4 (3 hours later) Time: _____
Water = 16 oz. (must be completely consumed prior to eating)
Write down all foods consumed:

_____

_____

_____

_____

_____

Meal #5 (3 hours later) Time: _____
Water = 16 oz. (must be completely consumed prior to eating)
Write down all foods consumed:

_____

_____

_____

_____

_____

WEEK ONE: Achieve a healthy schedule of eating

DAY FOUR: _____

WEEK ONE INTENTION (Repeat aloud 5 times in the morning and 5 times at night. Repeat silently 3 times prior to each meal):
I CREATE HEALTHY HABITS FOR MYSELF (AND MY FAMILY)

Meal #1 (within one hour of awakening) Time: _____
Water = 16 oz. (must be completely consumed prior to eating)
Write down all foods consumed:

_____

_____

_____

_____

Meal #2 (3 hours later) Time: _____
Water = 16 oz. (must be completely consumed prior to eating)
Write down all foods consumed:

_____

_____

_____

_____

Meal #3 (3 hours later) Time: _____
Water = 16 oz. (must be completely consumed prior to eating)
Write down all foods consumed:

_____

_____

_____

_____

Meal #4 (3 hours later) Time: _____
Water = 16 oz. (must be completely consumed prior to eating)
Write down all foods consumed:

_____

_____

_____

_____

_____

Meal #5 (3 hours later) Time: _____
Water = 16 oz. (must be completely consumed prior to eating)
Write down all foods consumed:

_____

_____

_____

_____

_____

WEEK ONE: Achieve a healthy schedule of eating

DAY FIVE: _____

WEEK ONE INTENTION (Repeat aloud 5 times in the morning and 5 times at night. Repeat silently 3 times prior to each meal):

I CREATE HEALTHY HABITS FOR MYSELF (AND MY FAMILY)

Meal #1 (within one hour of awakening) Time: _____
Water = 16 oz. (must be completely consumed prior to eating)
Write down all foods consumed:

_____

_____

_____

_____

Meal #2 (3 hours later) Time: _____
Water = 16 oz. (must be completely consumed prior to eating)
Write down all foods consumed:

_____

_____

_____

_____

Meal #3 (3 hours later) Time: _____
Water = 16 oz. (must be completely consumed prior to eating)
Write down all foods consumed:

_____

_____

_____

_____

Meal #4 (3 hours later) Time: _____
Water = 16 oz. (must be completely consumed prior to eating)
Write down all foods consumed:

_____

_____

_____

_____

_____

Meal #5 (3 hours later) Time: _____
Water = 16 oz. (must be completely consumed prior to eating)
Write down all foods consumed:

_____

_____

_____

_____

_____

WEEK ONE: Achieve a healthy schedule of eating

DAY SIX: _____

WEEK ONE INTENTION (Repeat aloud 5 times in the morning and 5 times at night. Repeat silently 3 times prior to each meal):

I CREATE HEALTHY HABITS FOR MYSELF (AND MY FAMILY)

Meal #1 (within one hour of awakening) Time: _____
Water = 16 oz. (must be completely consumed prior to eating)
Write down all foods consumed:

_____

_____

_____

_____

Meal #2 (3 hours later) Time: _____
Water = 16 oz. (must be completely consumed prior to eating)
Write down all foods consumed:

_____

_____

_____

_____

Meal #3 (3 hours later) Time: _____
Water = 16 oz. (must be completely consumed prior to eating)
Write down all foods consumed:

_____

_____

_____

_____

Meal #4 (3 hours later) Time: _____
Water = 16 oz. (must be completely consumed prior to eating)
Write down all foods consumed:

_____

_____

_____

_____

_____

Meal #5 (3 hours later) Time: _____
Water = 16 oz. (must be completely consumed prior to eating)
Write down all foods consumed:

_____

_____

_____

_____

_____

WEEK ONE: Achieve a healthy schedule of eating

DAY SEVEN: _____

WEEK ONE INTENTION (Repeat aloud 5 times in the morning and 5 times at night. Repeat silently 3 times prior to each meal):

I CREATE HEALTHY HABITS FOR MYSELF (AND MY FAMILY)

Meal #1 (within one hour of awakening) Time: _____

Water = 16 oz. (must be completely consumed prior to eating)

Write down all foods consumed:

_____

_____

_____

_____

Meal #2 (3 hours later) Time: _____

Water = 16 oz. (must be completely consumed prior to eating)

Write down all foods consumed:

_____

_____

_____

_____

Meal #3 (3 hours later) Time: _____

Water = 16 oz. (must be completely consumed prior to eating)

Write down all foods consumed:

_____

_____

_____

_____

Meal #4 (3 hours later) Time: _____
Water = 16 oz. (must be completely consumed prior to eating)
Write down all foods consumed:

_____

_____

_____

_____

_____

Meal #5 (3 hours later) Time: _____
Water = 16 oz. (must be completely consumed prior to eating)
Write down all foods consumed:

_____

_____

_____

_____

_____

WEEK TWO: Achieve a stronger body

Now that you have established what may be the most difficult part of the Plan – systematic eating – you are ready to begin to build the healthy baseline. We start with the very important macronutrient, protein. Protein is necessary for muscle tissue building and repair. You cannot make your exercise work for you without adequate protein.

The Plan focuses only on animal proteins because they are more readily assimilated by the body and better support strength gains through the exercises that I will provide you (if applicable). This is not to say that if you are vegan, you cannot succeed with the Plan. On the contrary – you absolutely can – you can simply make the adjustment in the protein choices and quantities. If you desire to follow a vegan or vegetarian Plan, I encourage you to coach with me. My website is http://www.achievelean.net.

The suggested protein choices listed in each meal all offer the required 20 grams of protein. You have the option to find an alternative protein to eat. Be sure it is an animal derived and that you are consuming 20 grams.

If you have been consuming inadequate amounts of protein throughout your day, the increased protein will make you feel fuller and possibly thicker. This is normal. Protein breaks down more slowly than carbohydrates and fibrous foods; hence the fuller feeling. You may immediately increase muscle tissue, which is necessary and important. However, while your body fat percentage is higher than desirable, the increase in muscle tissue results in thickness. Your measurements may reflect the thickening. Do not dismay! In a very short time as your body fat composition changes, the thickness will turn to lean.

As a side note, if you are training with me, you will likely begin to see a decrease in measurements with the added protein, and not the thickening, because I have designed the exercise programs to accommodate this caloric increase.

To sum up, by the end of Week Two, you will have established:

- Increased protein consumption
- Improved quality of protein consumed
- Increased strength, flexibility and functional movement as a result of lean mass gains

WEEK TWO: Achieve a stronger body
DAY ONE: _____

WEEK TWO INTENTION (Repeat aloud 5 times in the morning and 5 times at night. Repeat silently 3 times prior to each meal):

I REJECT UNHEALTHY HABITS

Abdomen msmt: _____   **Waist msmt:** _____   **Hip msmt:** _____

Meal #1 (within one hour of awakening) Time: _____
Water = 16 oz. (must be completely consumed prior to eating)
ADD:
Protein = 20g **Choose one:**   1 cup plain Greek yogurt   3 eggs
1-2 scoop protein powder mixed w/ 20 oz. water
Alternate protein: _____

LIST all other foods consumed:

_____

_____

_____

Meal #2 (3 hours later) Time: _____
Water = 16 oz. (must be completely consumed prior to eating)
ADD:
Protein = 20g **Choose one:**   ¾ cup cottage cheese   ½ can tuna
Alternate protein: _____

LIST all other foods consumed:

_____

_____

_____

Meal #3 (3 hours later) Time: _____
Water = 16 oz. (must be completely consumed prior to eating)
ADD:
Protein = 20g **Choose one:**   ¾ cup cottage cheese
3 oz. grass-fed beef, chicken breast or pork
Alternate protein: _____

LIST all other foods consumed:

_____

_____

_____

Meal #4 (3 hours later) Time: _____
Water = 16 oz. (must be completely consumed prior to eating)
ADD:
Protein = 20g **Choose one:**   1cup plain Greek yogurt
6 oz. wild caught fresh fish   3 oz. grass-fed beef, chicken breast or pork
1-2 scoop protein powder mixed w/ 20 oz. water
Alternate protein: _____

LIST all other foods consumed:

_____

_____

_____

Meal #5 (3 hours later) Time: _____
Water = 16 oz. (must be completely consumed prior to eating)
ADD:
Protein = 20g **Choose one:**   6 oz. wild caught fresh fish
3 oz. grass-fed beef, chicken breast or pork
Alternate protein: _____

LIST all other foods consumed:

_____

_____

_____

WEEK TWO: Achieve a stronger body

DAY TWO: _____

WEEK TWO INTENTION (Repeat aloud 5 times in the morning and 5 times at night. Repeat silently 3 times prior to each meal):

Meal #1 (within one hour of awakening) Time: _____

Water = 16 oz. (must be completely consumed prior to eating)

ADD:

Protein = 20g **Choose one:**   1 cup plain Greek yogurt   3 eggs

1-2 scoop protein powder mixed w/ 20 oz. water

Alternate protein: _____

LIST all other foods consumed:

_____

_____

_____

Meal #2 (3 hours later) Time: _____

Water = 16 oz. (must be completely consumed prior to eating)

ADD:

Protein = 20g **Choose one:**   ¾ cup cottage cheese   ½ can tuna

Alternate protein: _____

LIST all other foods consumed:

_____

_____

_____

Meal #3 (3 hours later) Time: _____

Water = 16 oz. (must be completely consumed prior to eating)

ADD:

Protein = 20g **Choose one:**   ¾ cup cottage cheese

3 oz. grass-fed beef, chicken breast or pork

Alternate protein: _____

LIST all other foods consumed:

_____

_____

_____

Meal #4 (3 hours later) Time: _____

Water = 16 oz. (must be completely consumed prior to eating)

ADD:

Protein = 20g **Choose one:**   1cup plain Greek yogurt

6 oz. wild caught fresh fish   3 oz. grass-fed beef, chicken breast or pork

1-2 scoop protein powder mixed w/ 20 oz. water

Alternate protein: _____

LIST all other foods consumed:

_____

_____

_____

Meal #5 (3 hours later) Time: _____

Water = 16 oz. (must be completely consumed prior to eating)

ADD:

Protein = 20g **Choose one:**   6 oz. wild caught fresh fish

3 oz. grass-fed beef, chicken breast or pork

Alternate protein: _____

LIST all other foods consumed:

_____

_____

_____

WEEK TWO: Achieve a stronger body
DAY THREE: _____

WEEK TWO INTENTION (Repeat aloud 5 times in the morning and 5 times at night. Repeat silently 3 times prior to each meal):

I REJECT UNHEALTHY HABITS

# Meal #1 (within one hour of awakening) Time: _____
Water = 16 oz. (must be completely consumed prior to eating)
ADD:
Protein = 20g **Choose one:**   1 cup plain Greek yogurt   3 eggs
1-2 scoop protein powder mixed w/ 20 oz. water
Alternate protein: _____

LIST all other foods consumed:

_____

_____

_____

# Meal #2 (3 hours later) Time: _____
Water = 16 oz. (must be completely consumed prior to eating)
ADD:
Protein = 20g **Choose one:**   ¾ cup cottage cheese   ½ can tuna
Alternate protein: _____

LIST all other foods consumed:

_____

_____

_____

Meal #3 (3 hours later) Time: _____

Water = 16 oz. (must be completely consumed prior to eating)

ADD:

Protein = 20g **Choose one:**   ¾ cup cottage cheese

3 oz. grass-fed beef, chicken breast or pork

Alternate protein: _____

LIST all other foods consumed:

_____

_____

_____

Meal #4 (3 hours later) Time: _____

Water = 16 oz. (must be completely consumed prior to eating)

ADD:

Protein = 20g **Choose one:**   1cup plain Greek yogurt

6 oz. wild caught fresh fish   3 oz. grass-fed beef, chicken breast or pork

1-2 scoop protein powder mixed w/ 20 oz. water

Alternate protein: _____

LIST all other foods consumed:

_____

_____

_____

Meal #5 (3 hours later) Time: _____

Water = 16 oz. (must be completely consumed prior to eating)

ADD:

Protein = 20g **Choose one:**   6 oz. wild caught fresh fish

3 oz. grass-fed beef, chicken breast or pork

Alternate protein: _____

LIST all other foods consumed:

_____

_____

_____

WEEK TWO: Achieve a stronger body
DAY FOUR: _____

WEEK TWO INTENTION (Repeat aloud 5 times in the morning and 5 times at night. Repeat silently 3 times prior to each meal):
I REJECT UNHEALTHY HABITS

# Meal #1 (within one hour of awakening) Time: _____
Water = 16 oz. (must be completely consumed prior to eating)
ADD:
Protein = 20g **Choose one:**   1 cup plain Greek yogurt   3 eggs
1-2 scoop protein powder mixed w/ 20 oz. water
Alternate protein: _____

LIST all other foods consumed:

_____

_____

_____

# Meal #2 (3 hours later) Time: _____
Water = 16 oz. (must be completely consumed prior to eating)
ADD:
Protein = 20g **Choose one:**   ¾ cup cottage cheese   ½ can tuna
Alternate protein: _____

LIST all other foods consumed:

_____

_____

_____

Meal #3 (3 hours later) Time: _____

Water = 16 oz. (must be completely consumed prior to eating)

ADD:

Protein = 20g **Choose one:**   ¾ cup cottage cheese

3 oz. grass-fed beef, chicken breast or pork

Alternate protein: _____

LIST all other foods consumed:

_____

_____

_____

Meal #4 (3 hours later) Time: _____

Water = 16 oz. (must be completely consumed prior to eating)

ADD:

Protein = 20g **Choose one:**   1cup plain Greek yogurt

6 oz. wild caught fresh fish   3 oz. grass-fed beef, chicken breast or pork

1-2 scoop protein powder mixed w/ 20 oz. water

Alternate protein: _____

LIST all other foods consumed:

_____

_____

_____

Meal #5 (3 hours later) Time: _____

Water = 16 oz. (must be completely consumed prior to eating)

ADD:

Protein = 20g **Choose one:**   6 oz. wild caught fresh fish

3 oz. grass-fed beef, chicken breast or pork

Alternate protein: _____

LIST all other foods consumed:

_____

_____

_____

WEEK TWO: Achieve a stronger body
DAY FIVE: _____

WEEK TWO INTENTION (Repeat aloud 5 times in the morning and 5 times at night. Repeat silently 3 times prior to each meal):
I REJECT UNHEALTHY HABITS

Meal #1 (within one hour of awakening) Time: _____
Water = 16 oz. (must be completely consumed prior to eating)
ADD:
Protein = 20g **Choose one:**   1 cup plain Greek yogurt   3 eggs
1-2 scoop protein powder mixed w/ 20 oz. water
Alternate protein: _____

LIST all other foods consumed:

_____

_____

_____

Meal #2 (3 hours later) Time: _____
Water = 16 oz. (must be completely consumed prior to eating)
ADD:
Protein = 20g **Choose one:**   ¾ cup cottage cheese   ½ can tuna
Alternate protein: _____

LIST all other foods consumed:

_____

_____

_____

Meal #3 (3 hours later) Time: _____
Water = 16 oz. (must be completely consumed prior to eating)
ADD:
Protein = 20g **Choose one:**   ¾ cup cottage cheese
3 oz. grass-fed beef, chicken breast or pork
Alternate protein: _____

LIST all other foods consumed:

_____

_____

_____

Meal #4 (3 hours later) Time: _____
Water = 16 oz. (must be completely consumed prior to eating)
ADD:
Protein = 20g **Choose one:**   1cup plain Greek yogurt
6 oz. wild caught fresh fish   3 oz. grass-fed beef, chicken breast or pork
1-2 scoop protein powder mixed w/ 20 oz. water
Alternate protein: _____

LIST all other foods consumed:

_____

_____

_____

Meal #5 (3 hours later) Time: _____
Water = 16 oz. (must be completely consumed prior to eating)
ADD:
Protein = 20g **Choose one:**   6 oz. wild caught fresh fish
3 oz. grass-fed beef, chicken breast or pork
Alternate protein: _____

LIST all other foods consumed:

_____

_____

_____

WEEK TWO: Achieve a stronger body
DAY SIX: _____

WEEK TWO INTENTION (Repeat aloud 5 times in the morning and 5 times at night. Repeat silently 3 times prior to each meal):

# Meal #1 (within one hour of awakening) Time: _____
Water = 16 oz. (must be completely consumed prior to eating)
ADD:
Protein = 20g **Choose one:**   1 cup plain Greek yogurt   3 eggs
1-2 scoop protein powder mixed w/ 20 oz. water
Alternate protein: _____

LIST all other foods consumed:

_____

_____

_____

# Meal #2 (3 hours later) Time: _____
Water = 16 oz. (must be completely consumed prior to eating)
ADD:
Protein = 20g **Choose one:**   ¾ cup cottage cheese   ½ can tuna
Alternate protein: _____

LIST all other foods consumed:

_____

_____

_____

Meal #3 (3 hours later) Time: _____

Water = 16 oz. (must be completely consumed prior to eating)

ADD:

Protein = 20g **Choose one:**   ¾ cup cottage cheese

3 oz. grass-fed beef, chicken breast or pork

Alternate protein: _____

LIST all other foods consumed:

_____

_____

_____

Meal #4 (3 hours later) Time: _____

Water = 16 oz. (must be completely consumed prior to eating)

ADD:

Protein = 20g **Choose one:**   1cup plain Greek yogurt

6 oz. wild caught fresh fish   3 oz. grass-fed beef, chicken breast or pork

1-2 scoop protein powder mixed w/ 20 oz. water

Alternate protein: _____

LIST all other foods consumed:

_____

_____

_____

Meal #5 (3 hours later) Time: _____

Water = 16 oz. (must be completely consumed prior to eating)

ADD:

Protein = 20g **Choose one:**   6 oz. wild caught fresh fish

3 oz. grass-fed beef, chicken breast or pork

Alternate protein: _____

LIST all other foods consumed:

_____

_____

_____

WEEK TWO: Achieve a stronger body
DAY SEVEN: _____

WEEK TWO INTENTION (Repeat aloud 5 times in the morning and 5 times at night. Repeat silently 3 times prior to each meal):

I REJECT UNHEALTHY HABITS

# Meal #1 (within one hour of awakening) Time: _____
Water = 16 oz. (must be completely consumed prior to eating)
ADD:
Protein = 20g **Choose one:**   1 cup plain Greek yogurt   3 eggs
1-2 scoop protein powder mixed w/ 20 oz. water
Alternate protein: _____

LIST all other foods consumed:

_____

_____

_____

# Meal #2 (3 hours later) Time: _____
Water = 16 oz. (must be completely consumed prior to eating)
ADD:
Protein = 20g **Choose one:**   ¾ cup cottage cheese   ½ can tuna
Alternate protein: _____

LIST all other foods consumed:

_____

_____

_____

Meal #3 (3 hours later) Time: _____

Water = 16 oz. (must be completely consumed prior to eating)
ADD:

Protein = 20g **Choose one:**   ¾ cup cottage cheese
3 oz. grass-fed beef, chicken breast or pork
Alternate protein: _____

LIST all other foods consumed:

_____

_____

_____

Meal #4 (3 hours later) Time: _____

Water = 16 oz. (must be completely consumed prior to eating)
ADD:

Protein = 20g **Choose one:**   1 cup plain Greek yogurt
6 oz. wild caught fresh fish   3 oz. grass-fed beef, chicken breast or pork
1-2 scoop protein powder mixed w/ 20 oz. water
Alternate protein: _____

LIST all other foods consumed:

_____

_____

_____

Meal #5 (3 hours later) Time: _____

Water = 16 oz. (must be completely consumed prior to eating)
ADD:

Protein = 20g **Choose one:**   6 oz. wild caught fresh fish
3 oz. grass-fed beef, chicken breast or pork
Alternate protein: _____

LIST all other foods consumed:

_____

_____

_____

WEEK THREE: Achieve a healthier digestive system

In Week Three we begin establishing metabolic health. Many of us are unable to improve our body composition because our metabolisms are unhealthy. In order to regain a healthy metabolism, we have to first address the digestive system, which must be clean and functional. Regular, healthy bowel movements are reflective of a healthy digestive tract and, ultimately, healthy metabolic activity.

We introduce fish oil capsules three times daily to improve metabolic performance. Please follow the recommended dosage of EPA and DHA so that you are receiving the full benefit of the fish oil. It is recommended that you choose capsules that are comprised of fats from sardines, anchovies, salmon and mackerel. You do not have to spend a lot on the capsules. They are readily available in stores and online for reasonable prices. They vary in quality and quantity of fatty acids – be sure to read the label and purchase accordingly.

We add a piece of fruit and non-digestible fiber in the first meal, vegetables and vegetable substitutes with every subsequent meal. Be sure to continue with the water consumption to assist with easy digestion and to diminish flatulence. Raw vegetables tend to be more difficult for the body to break down and therefore may not be as nutritionally valuable as lightly cooked vegetables. However, if you want to consume raw veggies for a meal or two, it will not deter from the baseline.

The vegetable substitutes are the non-digestible fibers – flax, wheat germ or dried greens – and nuts. If you have never ingested flax, wheat germ or dried greens, experiment with both palatability and gastric impact. If you have food sensitivities, the flax and wheat germ may not be ideal. The greens may be best served up in a blended protein shake with your fruit as they tend to have a very strong flavor.

Some of these foods will take time to like. Stick with the Plan and experiment with different ways of serving these foods. Flax and wheat germ are good mixed in yogurt, cottage cheese or oatmeal. You can mash a banana and mix it into plain yogurt with cinnamon and ground flax. Get creative and experiment with the choices provided. You will come up with something that is at least tolerable if not delicious!

To sum up, by the end of Week Three, you will have established:
- Increased fiber consumption in the form of fruit, vegetables and vegetable substitutes
- A healthier digestive system
- Improved energy and overall feelings of wellness
- Greater functional movement with decreased joint pain

WEEK THREE: Achieve a healthier digestive system
DAY ONE: _____

WEEK THREE INTENTION (Repeat aloud 5 times in the morning and 5 times at night. Repeat silently 3 times prior to each meal):

I AM HEALTHY AND STRONG

Abdomen msmt: _____   **Waist msmt:** _____   **Hip msmt:** _____

Meal #1 (within one hour of awakening)   **Time:** _____
Water = 16 oz. (must be completely consumed prior to eating)
Protein = 20g **Choose one:**   1 cup plain Greek yogurt   3 eggs
1-2 scoop protein powder mixed w/ 20 oz. water
Alternate protein: _____
ADD: Fruit = small to medium piece _____
Vegetable = 2 T flax, wheat germ, dried greens
 Fish Oil capsules = 2 @ 300 mg total combined EPA & DHA (from sardines, anchovies, salmon, mackerel)
LIST all other foods consumed:

_____

_____

Meal #2 (3 hours later)   **Time:** _____
Water = 16 oz. (must be completely consumed prior to eating)
Protein = 20g **Choose one:**   ¾ cup cottage cheese   ½ can tuna
Alternate protein: _____
ADD: Vegetable = 1 serving fresh or frozen – lightly steamed, roasted or baked
LIST all other foods consumed:

_____

_____

Meal #3 (3 hours later) **Time:** _____

Water = 16 oz. (must be completely consumed prior to eating)

Protein = 20g **Choose one:**   ¾ cup cottage cheese

3 oz. grass-fed beef, chicken breast or pork

Alternate protein: _____

ADD:

Vegetable = 1-2 servings fresh or frozen – lightly steamed, roasted or baked

Fish Oil capsules = 2 @ 300 mg total combined EPA & DHA (from sardines, anchovies, salmon, mackerel)

LIST all other foods consumed:

_____

_____

Meal #4 (3 hours later) **Time:** _____

Water = 16 oz. (must be completely consumed prior to eating)

Protein = 20g **Choose one:**   1 cup plain Greek yogurt

6 oz. wild caught fresh fish   3 oz. grass-fed beef, chicken breast or pork

1-2 scoop protein powder mixed w/ 20 oz. water

Alternate protein: _____

ADD:

Nuts = ¼ cup (almonds, brazil, pecans, walnuts) **OR**

Vegetable = 1 serving fresh or frozen – lightly steamed, roasted or baked

LIST all other foods consumed:

_____

_____

Meal #5 (3 hours later) **Time:** _____

Water = 16 oz. (must be completely consumed prior to eating)

Protein = 20g **Choose one:**   6 oz. wild caught fresh fish

3 oz. grass-fed beef, chicken breast or pork

Alternate protein: _____

ADD:

Vegetable = 2-3 servings fresh or frozen – lightly steamed, roasted or baked

Fish Oil capsules = 2 @ 300 mg total combined EPA & DHA (from sardines, anchovies, salmon, mackerel)

LIST all other foods consumed:

_____

_____

WEEK THREE: Achieve a healthier digestive system
DAY TWO: _____

WEEK THREE INTENTION (Repeat aloud 5 times in the morning and 5 times at night. Repeat silently 3 times prior to each meal):
I AM HEALTHY AND STRONG

Meal #1 (within one hour of awakening)   **Time:** _____
Water = 16 oz. (must be completely consumed prior to eating)
Protein = 20g **Choose one:**   1 cup plain Greek yogurt   3 eggs
1-2 scoop protein powder mixed w/ 20 oz. water
Alternate protein: _____
ADD: Fruit = small to medium piece _____
Vegetable = 2 T flax, wheat germ, dried greens
 Fish Oil capsules = 2 @ 300 mg total combined EPA & DHA (from sardines, anchovies, salmon, mackerel)
LIST all other foods consumed:

_____

_____

Meal #2 (3 hours later) **Time:** _____
Water = 16 oz. (must be completely consumed prior to eating)
Protein = 20g **Choose one:**   ¾ cup cottage cheese   ½ can tuna
Alternate protein: _____
ADD: Vegetable = 1 serving fresh or frozen – lightly steamed, roasted or baked
LIST all other foods consumed:

_____

_____

Meal #3 (3 hours later) **Time:** _____

Water = 16 oz. (must be completely consumed prior to eating)

Protein = 20g **Choose one:**   ¾ cup cottage cheese

3 oz. grass-fed beef, chicken breast or pork

Alternate protein: _____

ADD:

Vegetable = 1-2 servings fresh or frozen – lightly steamed, roasted or baked

Fish Oil capsules = 2 @ 300 mg total combined EPA & DHA (from sardines, anchovies, salmon, mackerel)

LIST all other foods consumed:

_____

_____

Meal #4 (3 hours later) **Time:** _____

Water = 16 oz. (must be completely consumed prior to eating)

Protein = 20g **Choose one:**   1cup plain Greek yogurt

6 oz. wild caught fresh fish   3 oz. grass-fed beef, chicken breast or pork

1-2 scoop protein powder mixed w/ 20 oz. water

Alternate protein: _____

ADD:

Nuts = ¼ cup (almonds, brazil, pecans, walnuts) **OR**

Vegetable = 1 serving fresh or frozen – lightly steamed, roasted or baked

LIST all other foods consumed:

_____

_____

Meal #5 (3 hours later) **Time:** _____

Water = 16 oz. (must be completely consumed prior to eating)

Protein = 20g **Choose one:**   6 oz. wild caught fresh fish

3 oz. grass-fed beef, chicken breast or pork

Alternate protein: _____

ADD:

Vegetable = 2-3 servings fresh or frozen – lightly steamed, roasted or baked

Fish Oil capsules = 2 @ 300 mg total combined EPA & DHA (from sardines, anchovies, salmon, mackerel)

LIST all other foods consumed:

_____

_____

WEEK THREE: Achieve a healthier digestive system
DAY THREE: _____

WEEK THREE INTENTION (Repeat aloud 5 times in the morning and 5 times at night. Repeat silently 3 times prior to each meal):

I AM HEALTHY AND STRONG

Meal #1 (within one hour of awakening)   **Time:** _____
Water = 16 oz. (must be completely consumed prior to eating)
Protein = 20g **Choose one:**   1 cup plain Greek yogurt   3 eggs
1-2 scoop protein powder mixed w/ 20 oz. water
Alternate protein: _____
ADD: Fruit = small to medium piece _____
Vegetable = 2 T flax, wheat germ, dried greens
 Fish Oil capsules = 2 @ 300 mg total combined EPA & DHA (from sardines, anchovies, salmon, mackerel)
LIST all other foods consumed:

_____

_____

Meal #2 (3 hours later) **Time:** _____
Water = 16 oz. (must be completely consumed prior to eating)
Protein = 20g **Choose one:**   ¾ cup cottage cheese   ½ can tuna
Alternate protein: _____
ADD: Vegetable = 1 serving fresh or frozen – lightly steamed, roasted or baked
LIST all other foods consumed:

_____

_____

Meal #3 (3 hours later) **Time:** _____

Water = 16 oz. (must be completely consumed prior to eating)

Protein = 20g **<u>Choose one:</u>**   ¾ cup cottage cheese

3 oz. grass-fed beef, chicken breast or pork

Alternate protein: _____

ADD:

Vegetable = 1-2 servings fresh or frozen – lightly steamed, roasted or baked

Fish Oil capsules = 2 @ 300 mg total combined EPA & DHA (from sardines, anchovies, salmon, mackerel)

LIST all other foods consumed:

_____

_____

Meal #4 (3 hours later) **Time:** _____

Water = 16 oz. (must be completely consumed prior to eating)

Protein = 20g **<u>Choose one:</u>**   1cup plain Greek yogurt

6 oz. wild caught fresh fish   3 oz. grass-fed beef, chicken breast or pork

1-2 scoop protein powder mixed w/ 20 oz. water

Alternate protein: _____

ADD:

Nuts = ¼ cup (almonds, brazil, pecans, walnuts) **OR**

Vegetable = 1 serving fresh or frozen – lightly steamed, roasted or baked

LIST all other foods consumed:

_____

_____

Meal #5 (3 hours later) **Time:** _____

Water = 16 oz. (must be completely consumed prior to eating)

Protein = 20g **<u>Choose one:</u>**   6 oz. wild caught fresh fish

3 oz. grass-fed beef, chicken breast or pork

Alternate protein: _____

ADD:

Vegetable = 2-3 servings fresh or frozen – lightly steamed, roasted or baked

Fish Oil capsules = 2 @ 300 mg total combined EPA & DHA (from sardines, anchovies, salmon, mackerel)

LIST all other foods consumed:

_____

_____

WEEK THREE: Achieve a healthier digestive system
DAY FOUR: _____

WEEK THREE INTENTION (Repeat aloud 5 times in the morning and 5 times at night. Repeat silently 3 times prior to each meal):

I AM HEALTHY AND STRONG

Meal #1 (within one hour of awakening)   Time: _____
Water = 16 oz. (must be completely consumed prior to eating)
Protein = 20g **Choose one:**   1 cup plain Greek yogurt   3 eggs
1-2 scoop protein powder mixed w/ 20 oz. water
Alternate protein: _____
ADD: Fruit = small to medium piece _____
Vegetable = 2 T flax, wheat germ, dried greens
 Fish Oil capsules = 2 @ 300 mg total combined EPA & DHA (from sardines, anchovies, salmon, mackerel)
LIST all other foods consumed:

_____

_____

Meal #2 (3 hours later) Time: _____
Water = 16 oz. (must be completely consumed prior to eating)
Protein = 20g **Choose one:**   ¾ cup cottage cheese   ½ can tuna
Alternate protein: _____
ADD: Vegetable = 1 serving fresh or frozen – lightly steamed, roasted or baked
LIST all other foods consumed:

_____

_____

Meal #3 (3 hours later)   **Time:** _____

Water = 16 oz. (must be completely consumed prior to eating)

Protein = 20g **Choose one:**   ¾ cup cottage cheese

3 oz. grass-fed beef, chicken breast or pork

Alternate protein: _____

ADD:

Vegetable = 1-2 servings fresh or frozen – lightly steamed, roasted or baked

Fish Oil capsules = 2 @ 300 mg total combined EPA & DHA (from sardines, anchovies, salmon, mackerel)

LIST all other foods consumed:

_____

_____

Meal #4 (3 hours later)   **Time:** _____

Water = 16 oz. (must be completely consumed prior to eating)

Protein = 20g **Choose one:**   1cup plain Greek yogurt

6 oz. wild caught fresh fish   3 oz. grass-fed beef, chicken breast or pork

1-2 scoop protein powder mixed w/ 20 oz. water

Alternate protein: _____

ADD:

Nuts = ¼ cup (almonds, brazil, pecans, walnuts) **OR**

Vegetable = 1 serving fresh or frozen – lightly steamed, roasted or baked

LIST all other foods consumed:

_____

_____

Meal #5 (3 hours later)   **Time:** _____

Water = 16 oz. (must be completely consumed prior to eating)

Protein = 20g **Choose one:**   6 oz. wild caught fresh fish

3 oz. grass-fed beef, chicken breast or pork

Alternate protein: _____

ADD:

Vegetable = 2-3 servings fresh or frozen – lightly steamed, roasted or baked

Fish Oil capsules = 2 @ 300 mg total combined EPA & DHA (from sardines, anchovies, salmon, mackerel)

LIST all other foods consumed:

_____

_____

WEEK THREE: Achieve a healthier digestive system
DAY FIVE: _____

WEEK THREE INTENTION (Repeat aloud 5 times in the morning and 5 times at night. Repeat silently 3 times prior to each meal):

I AM HEALTHY AND STRONG

Meal #1 (within one hour of awakening)   **Time:** _____
Water = 16 oz. (must be completely consumed prior to eating)
Protein = 20g **Choose one:**   1 cup plain Greek yogurt   3 eggs
1-2 scoop protein powder mixed w/ 20 oz. water
Alternate protein: _____
ADD: Fruit = small to medium piece _____
Vegetable = 2 T flax, wheat germ, dried greens
 Fish Oil capsules = 2 @ 300 mg total combined EPA & DHA (from sardines, anchovies, salmon, mackerel)
LIST all other foods consumed:

_____

_____

Meal #2 (3 hours later) **Time:** _____
Water = 16 oz. (must be completely consumed prior to eating)
Protein = 20g **Choose one:**   ¾ cup cottage cheese   ½ can tuna
Alternate protein: _____
ADD: Vegetable = 1 serving fresh or frozen – lightly steamed, roasted or baked
LIST all other foods consumed:

_____

_____

Meal #3 (3 hours later) **Time:** _____
Water = 16 oz. (must be completely consumed prior to eating)
Protein = 20g **Choose one:**   ¾ cup cottage cheese
3 oz. grass-fed beef, chicken breast or pork
Alternate protein: _____
ADD:
Vegetable = 1-2 servings fresh or frozen – lightly steamed, roasted or baked
Fish Oil capsules = 2 @ 300 mg total combined EPA & DHA (from sardines, anchovies, salmon, mackerel)
LIST all other foods consumed:

_____

_____

Meal #4 (3 hours later) **Time:** _____
Water = 16 oz. (must be completely consumed prior to eating)
Protein = 20g **Choose one:**   1cup plain Greek yogurt
6 oz. wild caught fresh fish   3 oz. grass-fed beef, chicken breast or pork
1-2 scoop protein powder mixed w/ 20 oz. water
Alternate protein: _____
ADD:
Nuts = ¼ cup (almonds, brazil, pecans, walnuts) **OR**
Vegetable = 1 serving fresh or frozen – lightly steamed, roasted or baked
LIST all other foods consumed:

_____

_____

Meal #5 (3 hours later) **Time:** _____
Water = 16 oz. (must be completely consumed prior to eating)
Protein = 20g **Choose one:**   6 oz. wild caught fresh fish
3 oz. grass-fed beef, chicken breast or pork
Alternate protein: _____
ADD:
Vegetable = 2-3 servings fresh or frozen – lightly steamed, roasted or baked
Fish Oil capsules = 2 @ 300 mg total combined EPA & DHA (from sardines, anchovies, salmon, mackerel)
LIST all other foods consumed:

_____

_____

WEEK THREE: Achieve a healthier digestive system
DAY SIX: _____

WEEK THREE INTENTION (Repeat aloud 5 times in the morning and 5 times at night. Repeat silently 3 times prior to each meal):

Meal #1 (within one hour of awakening)   **Time:** _____
Water = 16 oz. (must be completely consumed prior to eating)
Protein = 20g **Choose one:**   1 cup plain Greek yogurt   3 eggs
1-2 scoop protein powder mixed w/ 20 oz. water
Alternate protein: _____
ADD: Fruit = small to medium piece _____
Vegetable = 2 T flax, wheat germ, dried greens
 Fish Oil capsules = 2 @ 300 mg total combined EPA & DHA (from sardines, anchovies, salmon, mackerel)
LIST all other foods consumed:

_____

_____

Meal #2 (3 hours later) **Time:** _____
Water = 16 oz. (must be completely consumed prior to eating)
Protein = 20g **Choose one:**   ¾ cup cottage cheese   ½ can tuna
Alternate protein: _____
ADD: Vegetable = 1 serving fresh or frozen – lightly steamed, roasted or baked
LIST all other foods consumed:

_____

_____

Meal #3 (3 hours later) **Time:** _____
Water = 16 oz. (must be completely consumed prior to eating)
Protein = 20g **Choose one:**   ¾ cup cottage cheese
3 oz. grass-fed beef, chicken breast or pork
Alternate protein: _____
ADD:
Vegetable = 1-2 servings fresh or frozen – lightly steamed, roasted or baked
Fish Oil capsules = 2 @ 300 mg total combined EPA & DHA (from sardines,
anchovies, salmon, mackerel)
LIST all other foods consumed:

_____

_____

Meal #4 (3 hours later) **Time:** _____
Water = 16 oz. (must be completely consumed prior to eating)
Protein = 20g **Choose one:**   1cup plain Greek yogurt
6 oz. wild caught fresh fish   3 oz. grass-fed beef, chicken breast or pork
1-2 scoop protein powder mixed w/ 20 oz. water
Alternate protein: _____
ADD:
Nuts = ¼ cup (almonds, brazil, pecans, walnuts) **OR**
Vegetable = 1 serving fresh or frozen – lightly steamed, roasted or baked
LIST all other foods consumed:

_____

_____

Meal #5 (3 hours later) **Time:** _____
Water = 16 oz. (must be completely consumed prior to eating)
Protein = 20g **Choose one:**   6 oz. wild caught fresh fish
3 oz. grass-fed beef, chicken breast or pork
Alternate protein: _____
ADD:
Vegetable = 2-3 servings fresh or frozen – lightly steamed, roasted or baked
Fish Oil capsules = 2 @ 300 mg total combined EPA & DHA (from sardines,
anchovies, salmon, mackerel)
LIST all other foods consumed:

_____

_____

WEEK THREE: Achieve a healthier digestive system
DAY SEVEN: _____

WEEK THREE INTENTION (Repeat aloud 5 times in the morning and 5 times at night. Repeat silently 3 times prior to each meal):

I AM HEALTHY AND STRONG

Meal #1 (within one hour of awakening) **Time:** _____
Water = 16 oz. (must be completely consumed prior to eating)
Protein = 20g **Choose one:**   1 cup plain Greek yogurt   3 eggs
1-2 scoop protein powder mixed w/ 20 oz. water
Alternate protein: _____
ADD: Fruit = small to medium piece _____
Vegetable = 2 T flax, wheat germ, dried greens
 Fish Oil capsules = 2 @ 300 mg total combined EPA & DHA (from sardines, anchovies, salmon, mackerel)
LIST all other foods consumed:

_____

_____

Meal #2 (3 hours later) **Time:** _____
Water = 16 oz. (must be completely consumed prior to eating)
Protein = 20g **Choose one:**   ¾ cup cottage cheese   ½ can tuna
Alternate protein: _____
ADD: Vegetable = 1 serving fresh or frozen – lightly steamed, roasted or baked
LIST all other foods consumed:

_____

_____

Meal #3 (3 hours later) **Time:** _____

Water = 16 oz. (must be completely consumed prior to eating)

Protein = 20g **Choose one:**   ¾ cup cottage cheese

3 oz. grass-fed beef, chicken breast or pork

Alternate protein: _____

ADD:

Vegetable = 1-2 servings fresh or frozen – lightly steamed, roasted or baked

Fish Oil capsules = 2 @ 300 mg total combined EPA & DHA (from sardines, anchovies, salmon, mackerel)

LIST all other foods consumed:

_____

_____

Meal #4 (3 hours later) **Time:** _____

Water = 16 oz. (must be completely consumed prior to eating)

Protein = 20g **Choose one:**   1cup plain Greek yogurt

6 oz. wild caught fresh fish   3 oz. grass-fed beef, chicken breast or pork

1-2 scoop protein powder mixed w/ 20 oz. water

Alternate protein: _____

ADD:

Nuts = ¼ cup (almonds, brazil, pecans, walnuts) **OR**

Vegetable = 1 serving fresh or frozen – lightly steamed, roasted or baked

LIST all other foods consumed:

_____

_____

Meal #5 (3 hours later) **Time:** _____

Water = 16 oz. (must be completely consumed prior to eating)

Protein = 20g **Choose one:**   6 oz. wild caught fresh fish

3 oz. grass-fed beef, chicken breast or pork

Alternate protein: _____

ADD:

Vegetable = 2-3 servings fresh or frozen – lightly steamed, roasted or baked

Fish Oil capsules = 2 @ 300 mg total combined EPA & DHA (from sardines, anchovies, salmon, mackerel)

LIST all other foods consumed:

_____

WEEK FOUR: Achieve cleaner eating

In Week Four we begin the gentle process of cleaning up the diet and subtracting unnecessary foods. Take this process as slowly as needed. Remember the goal is to naturally change your attitude towards food, improve your awareness of food choices, and slowly change food preferences. You must not deprive. If you do, you will set yourself up for cravings, which will quickly throw you off the Plan. If you go through the entire Plan slowly, naturally decreasing unhealthy food choices, you will never feel deprived and will surely succeed.

The first meal is typically the easiest to minimize food quantity, so that is the first meal from which we subtract. You may not even be consuming extra foods at this time of day. Good. Follow the Plan and establish a healthy pattern of eating just enough but not too much in the morning.

Continue writing everything down. We are still in the process of creating awareness of food choices. Hopefully, you are spending a bit more time in the store reading label ingredients and learning more about the foods you purchase. Also, you may find you spend more time in the fresh produce section, the fresh meats and dairy sections, and less time in the middle isles, which typically have the packaged, processed foods. Good for you! Keep up the good work – you are half way through the Plan, and you will soon see dramatic changes in your measurements and in how you feel.

To sum up, by the end of Week Four, you will have established:
- Subtraction of unhealthy foods from at least the first meal of the day
- A stronger, healthier, and slightly leaner physique

WEEK FOUR: Achieve cleaner eating
DAY ONE: _____

WEEK FOUR INTENTION (Repeat aloud 5 times in the morning and 5 times at night. Repeat silently 3 times prior to each meal):

MY WILLPOWER IS STRONG AND I REJECT UNHEALTHY HABITS

Abdomen msmt: _____   **Waist msmt:** _____   **Hip msmt:** _____

# Meal #1 (within one hour of awakening) Time: _____
Water = 16 oz. (must be completely consumed prior to eating)
Protein = 20g **Choose one:**   1 cup plain Greek yogurt   3 eggs
1-2 scoop protein powder mixed w/ 20 oz. water
Alternate protein: _____
Fruit = small to medium piece _____
Vegetable = 2 T flax, wheat germ, dried greens
Fish Oil capsules = 2 @ 300 mg total combined EPA & DHA (from sardines, anchovies, salmon, mackerel)
NO additional foods consumed

# Meal #2 (3 hours later) Time: _____
Water = 16 oz. (must be completely consumed prior to eating)
Protein = 20g **Choose one:**   ¾ cup cottage cheese   ½ can tuna
Alternate protein: _____
Vegetable = 1 serving fresh or frozen – lightly steamed, roasted or baked
1 additional food item allowed:
_____

Meal #3 (3 hours later) **Time:** _____
Water = 16 oz. (must be completely consumed prior to eating)
Protein = 20g **Choose one:**   ¾ cup cottage cheese
3 oz. grass-fed beef, chicken breast or pork
Alternate protein: _____
Vegetable = 1-2 servings fresh or frozen – lightly steamed, roasted or baked
Fish Oil capsules = 2 @ 300 mg total combined EPA & DHA (from sardines,
anchovies, salmon, mackerel)
1 additional food item allowed:

_____

Meal #4 (3 hours later) **Time:** _____
Water = 16 oz. (must be completely consumed prior to eating)
Protein = 20g **Choose one:**   1cup plain Greek yogurt
6 oz. wild caught fresh fish   3 oz. grass-fed beef, chicken breast or pork
1-2 scoop protein powder mixed w/ 20 oz. water
Alternate protein: _____
ADD:
Nuts = ¼ cup (almonds, brazil, pecans, walnuts) **OR**
Vegetable = 1 serving fresh or frozen – lightly steamed, roasted or baked
1 additional food item allowed:

_____

Meal #5 (3 hours later) **Time:** _____
Water = 16 oz. (must be completely consumed prior to eating)
Protein = 20g **Choose one:**   6 oz. wild caught fresh fish
3 oz. grass-fed beef, chicken breast or pork
Alternate protein: _____
Vegetable = 2-3 servings fresh or frozen – lightly steamed, roasted or baked
Fish Oil capsules = 2 @ 300 mg total combined EPA & DHA (from sardines,
anchovies, salmon, mackerel)
1 additional food item allowed:

_____

WEEK FOUR: Achieve cleaner eating
DAY TWO: _____

WEEK FOUR INTENTION (Repeat aloud 5 times in the morning and 5 times at night. Repeat silently 3 times prior to each meal):

MY WILLPOWER IS STRONG AND I REJECT UNHEALTHY HABITS

Meal #1 (within one hour of awakening) **Time:** _____
Water = 16 oz. (must be completely consumed prior to eating)
Protein = 20g **Choose one:**   1 cup plain Greek yogurt   3 eggs
1-2 scoop protein powder mixed w/ 20 oz. water
Alternate protein: _____
Fruit = small to medium piece _____
Vegetable = 2 T flax, wheat germ, dried greens
Fish Oil capsules = 2 @ 300 mg total combined EPA & DHA (from sardines, anchovies, salmon, mackerel)
NO additional foods consumed

Meal #2 (3 hours later) **Time:** _____
Water = 16 oz. (must be completely consumed prior to eating)
Protein = 20g **Choose one:**   ¾ cup cottage cheese   ½ can tuna
Alternate protein: _____
Vegetable = 1 serving fresh or frozen – lightly steamed, roasted or baked
1 additional food item allowed:

_____

Meal #3 (3 hours later)   **Time:** _____

Water = 16 oz. (must be completely consumed prior to eating)

Protein = 20g **Choose one:**   ¾ cup cottage cheese

3 oz. grass-fed beef, chicken breast or pork

Alternate protein: _____

Vegetable = 1-2 servings fresh or frozen – lightly steamed, roasted or baked

Fish Oil capsules = 2 @ 300 mg total combined EPA & DHA (from sardines, anchovies, salmon, mackerel)

1 additional food item allowed:

_____

Meal #4 (3 hours later)   **Time:** _____

Water = 16 oz. (must be completely consumed prior to eating)

Protein = 20g **Choose one:**   1 cup plain Greek yogurt

6 oz. wild caught fresh fish   3 oz. grass-fed beef, chicken breast or pork

1-2 scoop protein powder mixed w/ 20 oz. water

Alternate protein: _____

ADD:

Nuts = ¼ cup (almonds, brazil, pecans, walnuts) **OR**

Vegetable = 1 serving fresh or frozen – lightly steamed, roasted or baked

1 additional food item allowed:

_____

Meal #5 (3 hours later)   **Time:** _____

Water = 16 oz. (must be completely consumed prior to eating)

Protein = 20g **Choose one:**   6 oz. wild caught fresh fish

3 oz. grass-fed beef, chicken breast or pork

Alternate protein: _____

Vegetable = 2-3 servings fresh or frozen – lightly steamed, roasted or baked

Fish Oil capsules = 2 @ 300 mg total combined EPA & DHA (from sardines, anchovies, salmon, mackerel)

1 additional food item allowed:

_____

WEEK FOUR: Achieve cleaner eating
DAY THREE: _____

WEEK FOUR INTENTION (Repeat aloud 5 times in the morning and 5 times at night. Repeat silently 3 times prior to each meal):
MY WILLPOWER IS STRONG AND I REJECT UNHEALTHY HABITS

# Meal #1 (within one hour of awakening) **Time:** _____
Water = 16 oz. (must be completely consumed prior to eating)
Protein = 20g **Choose one:**   1 cup plain Greek yogurt   3 eggs
1-2 scoop protein powder mixed w/ 20 oz. water
Alternate protein: _____
Fruit = small to medium piece _____
Vegetable = 2 T flax, wheat germ, dried greens
Fish Oil capsules = 2 @ 300 mg total combined EPA & DHA (from sardines, anchovies, salmon, mackerel)
NO additional foods consumed

# Meal #2 (3 hours later) **Time:** _____
Water = 16 oz. (must be completely consumed prior to eating)
Protein = 20g **Choose one:**   ¾ cup cottage cheese   ½ can tuna
Alternate protein: _____
Vegetable = 1 serving fresh or frozen – lightly steamed, roasted or baked
1 additional food item allowed:
_____

Meal #3 (3 hours later) **Time:** _____

Water = 16 oz. (must be completely consumed prior to eating)

Protein = 20g **Choose one:**   ¾ cup cottage cheese

3 oz. grass-fed beef, chicken breast or pork

Alternate protein: _____

Vegetable = 1-2 servings fresh or frozen – lightly steamed, roasted or baked

Fish Oil capsules = 2 @ 300 mg total combined EPA & DHA (from sardines, anchovies, salmon, mackerel)

1 additional food item allowed:

Meal #4 (3 hours later) **Time:** _____

Water = 16 oz. (must be completely consumed prior to eating)

Protein = 20g **Choose one:**   1 cup plain Greek yogurt

6 oz. wild caught fresh fish   3 oz. grass-fed beef, chicken breast or pork

1-2 scoop protein powder mixed w/ 20 oz. water

Alternate protein: _____

ADD:

Nuts = ¼ cup (almonds, brazil, pecans, walnuts) **OR**

Vegetable = 1 serving fresh or frozen – lightly steamed, roasted or baked

1 additional food item allowed:

Meal #5 (3 hours later) **Time:** _____

Water = 16 oz. (must be completely consumed prior to eating)

Protein = 20g **Choose one:**   6 oz. wild caught fresh fish

3 oz. grass-fed beef, chicken breast or pork

Alternate protein: _____

Vegetable = 2-3 servings fresh or frozen – lightly steamed, roasted or baked

Fish Oil capsules = 2 @ 300 mg total combined EPA & DHA (from sardines, anchovies, salmon, mackerel)

1 additional food item allowed:

WEEK FOUR: Achieve cleaner eating
DAY FOUR: _____

WEEK FOUR INTENTION (Repeat aloud 5 times in the morning and 5 times at night. Repeat silently 3 times prior to each meal):

MY WILLPOWER IS STRONG AND I REJECT UNHEALTHY HABITS

Meal #1 (within one hour of awakening)   Time: _____
Water = 16 oz. (must be completely consumed prior to eating)
Protein = 20g **Choose one:**   1 cup plain Greek yogurt   3 eggs
1-2 scoop protein powder mixed w/ 20 oz. water
Alternate protein: _____
Fruit = small to medium piece _____
Vegetable = 2 T flax, wheat germ, dried greens
Fish Oil capsules = 2 @ 300 mg total combined EPA & DHA (from sardines, anchovies, salmon, mackerel)
NO additional foods consumed

Meal #2 (3 hours later)   Time: _____
Water = 16 oz. (must be completely consumed prior to eating)
Protein = 20g **Choose one:**   ¾ cup cottage cheese   ½ can tuna
Alternate protein: _____
Vegetable = 1 serving fresh or frozen – lightly steamed, roasted or baked
1 additional food item allowed:
_____

Meal #3 (3 hours later) Time: _____

Water = 16 oz. (must be completely consumed prior to eating)
Protein = 20g **Choose one:**   ¾ cup cottage cheese
3 oz. grass-fed beef, chicken breast or pork
Alternate protein: _____
Vegetable = 1-2 servings fresh or frozen – lightly steamed, roasted or baked
Fish Oil capsules = 2 @ 300 mg total combined EPA & DHA (from sardines,
anchovies, salmon, mackerel)
1 additional food item allowed:

Meal #4 (3 hours later) Time: _____

Water = 16 oz. (must be completely consumed prior to eating)
Protein = 20g **Choose one:**   1cup plain Greek yogurt
6 oz. wild caught fresh fish   3 oz. grass-fed beef, chicken breast or pork
1-2 scoop protein powder mixed w/ 20 oz. water
Alternate protein: _____
ADD:
Nuts = ¼ cup (almonds, brazil, pecans, walnuts) **OR**
Vegetable = 1 serving fresh or frozen – lightly steamed, roasted or baked
1 additional food item allowed:

Meal #5 (3 hours later) Time: _____

Water = 16 oz. (must be completely consumed prior to eating)
Protein = 20g **Choose one:**   6 oz. wild caught fresh fish
3 oz. grass-fed beef, chicken breast or pork
Alternate protein: _____
Vegetable = 2-3 servings fresh or frozen – lightly steamed, roasted or baked
Fish Oil capsules = 2 @ 300 mg total combined EPA & DHA (from sardines,
anchovies, salmon, mackerel)
1 additional food item allowed:

WEEK FOUR: Achieve cleaner eating
DAY FIVE: _____

Meal #1 (within one hour of awakening)   Time: _____
Water = 16 oz. (must be completely consumed prior to eating)
Protein = 20g **Choose one:**   1 cup plain Greek yogurt   3 eggs
1-2 scoop protein powder mixed w/ 20 oz. water
Alternate protein: _____
Fruit = small to medium piece _____
Vegetable = 2 T flax, wheat germ, dried greens
Fish Oil capsules = 2 @ 300 mg total combined EPA & DHA (from sardines, anchovies, salmon, mackerel)
NO additional foods consumed

Meal #2 (3 hours later) Time: _____
Water = 16 oz. (must be completely consumed prior to eating)
Protein = 20g **Choose one:**   ¾ cup cottage cheese   ½ can tuna
Alternate protein: _____
Vegetable = 1 serving fresh or frozen – lightly steamed, roasted or baked
1 additional food item allowed:

_____

Meal #3 (3 hours later) **Time:** _____

Water = 16 oz. (must be completely consumed prior to eating)

Protein = 20g **Choose one:**   ¾ cup cottage cheese

3 oz. grass-fed beef, chicken breast or pork

Alternate protein: _____

Vegetable = 1-2 servings fresh or frozen – lightly steamed, roasted or baked

Fish Oil capsules = 2 @ 300 mg total combined EPA & DHA (from sardines, anchovies, salmon, mackerel)

1 additional food item allowed:

Meal #4 (3 hours later) **Time:** _____

Water = 16 oz. (must be completely consumed prior to eating)

Protein = 20g **Choose one:**   1 cup plain Greek yogurt

6 oz. wild caught fresh fish   3 oz. grass-fed beef, chicken breast or pork

1-2 scoop protein powder mixed w/ 20 oz. water

Alternate protein: _____

ADD:

Nuts = ¼ cup (almonds, brazil, pecans, walnuts) **OR**

Vegetable = 1 serving fresh or frozen – lightly steamed, roasted or baked

1 additional food item allowed:

Meal #5 (3 hours later) **Time:** _____

Water = 16 oz. (must be completely consumed prior to eating)

Protein = 20g **Choose one:**   6 oz. wild caught fresh fish

3 oz. grass-fed beef, chicken breast or pork

Alternate protein: _____

Vegetable = 2-3 servings fresh or frozen – lightly steamed, roasted or baked

Fish Oil capsules = 2 @ 300 mg total combined EPA & DHA (from sardines, anchovies, salmon, mackerel)

1 additional food item allowed:

WEEK FOUR: Achieve cleaner eating
DAY SIX: _____

WEEK FOUR INTENTION (Repeat aloud 5 times in the morning and 5 times at night. Repeat silently 3 times prior to each meal):

MY WILLPOWER IS STRONG AND I REJECT UNHEALTHY HABITS

Meal #1 (within one hour of awakening)   Time: _____
Water = 16 oz. (must be completely consumed prior to eating)
Protein = 20g **Choose one:**   1 cup plain Greek yogurt   3 eggs
1-2 scoop protein powder mixed w/ 20 oz. water
Alternate protein: _____
Fruit = small to medium piece _____
Vegetable = 2 T flax, wheat germ, dried greens
Fish Oil capsules = 2 @ 300 mg total combined EPA & DHA (from sardines, anchovies, salmon, mackerel)
NO additional foods consumed

Meal #2 (3 hours later)   Time: _____
Water = 16 oz. (must be completely consumed prior to eating)
Protein = 20g **Choose one:**   ¾ cup cottage cheese   ½ can tuna
Alternate protein: _____
Vegetable = 1 serving fresh or frozen – lightly steamed, roasted or baked
1 additional food item allowed:
_____

Meal #3 (3 hours later) **Time:** _____

Water = 16 oz. (must be completely consumed prior to eating)

Protein = 20g **Choose one:**   ¾ cup cottage cheese

3 oz. grass-fed beef, chicken breast or pork

Alternate protein: _____

Vegetable = 1-2 servings fresh or frozen – lightly steamed, roasted or baked

Fish Oil capsules = 2 @ 300 mg total combined EPA & DHA (from sardines, anchovies, salmon, mackerel)

1 additional food item allowed:

Meal #4 (3 hours later) **Time:** _____

Water = 16 oz. (must be completely consumed prior to eating)

Protein = 20g **Choose one:**   1 cup plain Greek yogurt

6 oz. wild caught fresh fish   3 oz. grass-fed beef, chicken breast or pork

1-2 scoop protein powder mixed w/ 20 oz. water

Alternate protein: _____

ADD:

Nuts = ¼ cup (almonds, brazil, pecans, walnuts) **OR**

Vegetable = 1 serving fresh or frozen – lightly steamed, roasted or baked

1 additional food item allowed:

Meal #5 (3 hours later) **Time:** _____

Water = 16 oz. (must be completely consumed prior to eating)

Protein = 20g **Choose one:**   6 oz. wild caught fresh fish

3 oz. grass-fed beef, chicken breast or pork

Alternate protein: _____

Vegetable = 2-3 servings fresh or frozen – lightly steamed, roasted or baked

Fish Oil capsules = 2 @ 300 mg total combined EPA & DHA (from sardines, anchovies, salmon, mackerel)

1 additional food item allowed:

WEEK FOUR: Achieve cleaner eating
DAY SEVEN: _____

WEEK FOUR INTENTION (Repeat aloud 5 times in the morning and 5 times at night. Repeat silently 3 times prior to each meal):

MY WILLPOWER IS STRONG AND I REJECT UNHEALTHY HABITS

# Meal #1 (within one hour of awakening)   Time: _____
Water = 16 oz. (must be completely consumed prior to eating)
Protein = 20g **Choose one:**   1 cup plain Greek yogurt   3 eggs
1-2 scoop protein powder mixed w/ 20 oz. water
Alternate protein: _____
Fruit = small to medium piece _____
Vegetable = 2 T flax, wheat germ, dried greens
Fish Oil capsules = 2 @ 300 mg total combined EPA & DHA (from sardines, anchovies, salmon, mackerel)
NO additional foods consumed

# Meal #2 (3 hours later)   Time: _____
Water = 16 oz. (must be completely consumed prior to eating)
Protein = 20g **Choose one:**   ¾ cup cottage cheese   ½ can tuna
Alternate protein: _____
Vegetable = 1 serving fresh or frozen – lightly steamed, roasted or baked
1 additional food item allowed:
_____

Meal #3 (3 hours later) **Time:** _____

Water = 16 oz. (must be completely consumed prior to eating)

Protein = 20g **Choose one:**   ¾ cup cottage cheese

3 oz. grass-fed beef, chicken breast or pork

Alternate protein: _____

Vegetable = 1-2 servings fresh or frozen – lightly steamed, roasted or baked

Fish Oil capsules = 2 @ 300 mg total combined EPA & DHA (from sardines, anchovies, salmon, mackerel)

1 additional food item allowed:

Meal #4 (3 hours later) **Time:** _____

Water = 16 oz. (must be completely consumed prior to eating)

Protein = 20g **Choose one:**   1cup plain Greek yogurt

6 oz. wild caught fresh fish   3 oz. grass-fed beef, chicken breast or pork

1-2 scoop protein powder mixed w/ 20 oz. water

Alternate protein: _____

ADD:

Nuts = ¼ cup (almonds, brazil, pecans, walnuts) **OR**

Vegetable = 1 serving fresh or frozen – lightly steamed, roasted or baked

1 additional food item allowed:

Meal #5 (3 hours later) **Time:** _____

Water = 16 oz. (must be completely consumed prior to eating)

Protein = 20g **Choose one:**   6 oz. wild caught fresh fish

3 oz. grass-fed beef, chicken breast or pork

Alternate protein: _____

Vegetable = 2-3 servings fresh or frozen – lightly steamed, roasted or baked

Fish Oil capsules = 2 @ 300 mg total combined EPA & DHA (from sardines, anchovies, salmon, mackerel)

1 additional food item allowed:

WEEK FIVE: Achieve healthy eating

Perhaps you have already begun subtracting the unhealthy, unnecessary foods from your diet naturally. If not, do not dismay. Approach Week Five with a strong conviction, and allow yourself to have setbacks. Take the entire week to achieve the eating as the Plan directs. And if you have to repeat Week Five, do it without regret. You should not move to Week Six until you are satisfied with your progress and comfortable with the subtraction of foods.

Continue to keep your food choice awareness high by writing down your meals as you consume them. Be patient and progress at a comfortable pace.

Once you master the Plan in Week Five, you will make remarkable progress. Stay with the Plan's progression so that you get the absolute best results from your efforts.

To sum up, by the end of Week Five, you will have established:
- Healthy eating habits
- Improved awareness of food choices
- A strong desire to succeed with the Plan

WEEK FIVE: Achieve healthy eating
DAY ONE: _____

WEEK FIVE INTENTION (Repeat aloud 5 times in the morning and 5 times at night. Repeat silently 3 times prior to each meal):
I SIMPLIFY

Abdomen msmt: _____   **Waist msmt:** _____   **Hip msmt:** _____

# Meal #1 (within one hour of awakening) **Time:** _____
Water = 16 oz. (must be completely consumed prior to eating)
Protein = 20g **Choose one:**   1 cup plain Greek yogurt   3 eggs
1-2 scoop protein powder mixed w/ 20 oz. water
Alternate protein: _____
Fruit = small to medium piece _____
Vegetable = 2 T flax, wheat germ, dried greens
Fish Oil capsules = 2 @ 300 mg total combined EPA & DHA (from sardines, anchovies, salmon, mackerel)

# Meal #2 (3 hours later) **Time:** _____
Water = 16 oz. (must be completely consumed prior to eating)
Protein = 20g **Choose one:**   ¾ cup cottage cheese   ½ can tuna
Alternate protein: _____
Vegetable = 1 serving fresh or frozen – lightly steamed, roasted or baked
NO additional foods consumed

# Meal #3 (3 hours later) **Time:** _____
Water = 16 oz. (must be completely consumed prior to eating)
Protein = 20g **Choose one:**   ¾ cup cottage cheese
3 oz. grass-fed beef, chicken breast or pork
Alternate protein: _____
Vegetable = 1-2 servings fresh or frozen – lightly steamed, roasted or baked
Fish Oil capsules = 2 @ 300 mg total combined EPA & DHA (from sardines, anchovies, salmon, mackerel)
1 additional food item allowed:

Meal #4 (3 hours later) **Time:** _____

Water = 16 oz. (must be completely consumed prior to eating)

Protein = 20g **Choose one:**   1cup plain Greek yogurt

6 oz. wild caught fresh fish3 oz. grass-fed beef, chicken breast or pork

1-2 scoop protein powder mixed w/ 20 oz. water

Alternate protein: _____

Nuts = ¼ cup (almonds, brazil, pecans, walnuts) **OR**

Vegetable = 1 serving fresh or frozen – lightly steamed, roasted or baked

NO additional foods consumed

Meal #5 (3 hours later) **Time:** _____

Water = 16 oz. (must be completely consumed prior to eating)

Protein = 20g **Choose one:**   6 oz. wild caught fresh fish

3 oz. grass-fed beef, chicken breast or pork

Alternate protein: _____

Vegetable = 2-3 servings fresh or frozen – lightly steamed, roasted or baked

Fish Oil capsules = 2 @ 300 mg total combined EPA & DHA (from sardines, anchovies, salmon, mackerel)

1 additional food item allowed:

_____

WEEK FIVE: Achieve healthy eating

DAY TWO: _____

WEEK FIVE INTENTION (Repeat aloud 5 times in the morning and 5 times at night. Repeat silently 3 times prior to each meal):

I SIMPLIFY

Meal #1 (within one hour of awakening) **Time:** _____

Water = 16 oz. (must be completely consumed prior to eating)

Protein = 20g **Choose one:**   1 cup plain Greek yogurt   3 eggs

1-2 scoop protein powder mixed w/ 20 oz. water

Alternate protein: _____

Fruit = small to medium piece _____

Vegetable = 2 T flax, wheat germ, dried greens

Fish Oil capsules = 2 @ 300 mg total combined EPA & DHA (from sardines, anchovies, salmon, mackerel)

Meal #2 (3 hours later) **Time:** _____

Water = 16 oz. (must be completely consumed prior to eating)

Protein = 20g **Choose one:**   ¾ cup cottage cheese   ½ can tuna

Alternate protein: _____

Vegetable = 1 serving fresh or frozen – lightly steamed, roasted or baked

NO additional foods consumed

Meal #3 (3 hours later) **Time:** _____

Water = 16 oz. (must be completely consumed prior to eating)

Protein = 20g **Choose one:**   ¾ cup cottage cheese

3 oz. grass-fed beef, chicken breast or pork

Alternate protein: _____

Vegetable = 1-2 servings fresh or frozen – lightly steamed, roasted or baked

Fish Oil capsules = 2 @ 300 mg total combined EPA & DHA (from sardines, anchovies, salmon, mackerel)

1 additional food item allowed:

Meal #4 (3 hours later)   Time: _____

Water = 16 oz. (must be completely consumed prior to eating)
Protein = 20g **Choose one:**   1cup plain Greek yogurt
6 oz. wild caught fresh fish 3 oz. grass-fed beef, chicken breast or pork
1-2 scoop protein powder mixed w/ 20 oz. water
Alternate protein: _____
Nuts = ¼ cup (almonds, brazil, pecans, walnuts) **OR**
Vegetable = 1 serving fresh or frozen – lightly steamed, roasted or baked
NO additional foods consumed

Meal #5 (3 hours later)   Time: _____

Water = 16 oz. (must be completely consumed prior to eating)
Protein = 20g **Choose one:**   6 oz. wild caught fresh fish
3 oz. grass-fed beef, chicken breast or pork
Alternate protein: _____
Vegetable = 2-3 servings fresh or frozen – lightly steamed, roasted or baked
Fish Oil capsules = 2 @ 300 mg total combined EPA & DHA (from sardines, anchovies, salmon, mackerel)
1 additional food item allowed:

_____

WEEK FIVE: Achieve healthy eating
DAY THREE: _____

WEEK FIVE INTENTION (Repeat aloud 5 times in the morning and 5 times at night. Repeat silently 3 times prior to each meal):
I SIMPLIFY

Meal #1 (within one hour of awakening) **Time:** _____
Water = 16 oz. (must be completely consumed prior to eating)
Protein = 20g **Choose one:**   1 cup plain Greek yogurt   3 eggs
1-2 scoop protein powder mixed w/ 20 oz. water
Alternate protein: _____
Fruit = small to medium piece ____ _____
Vegetable = 2 T flax, wheat germ, dried greens
Fish Oil capsules = 2 @ 300 mg total combined EPA & DHA (from sardines, anchovies, salmon, mackerel)

Meal #2 (3 hours later) **Time:** _____
Water = 16 oz. (must be completely consumed prior to eating)
Protein = 20g **Choose one:**   ¾ cup cottage cheese   ½ can tuna
Alternate protein: _____
Vegetable = 1 serving fresh or frozen – lightly steamed, roasted or baked
NO additional foods consumed

Meal #3 (3 hours later) **Time:** _____
Water = 16 oz. (must be completely consumed prior to eating)
Protein = 20g **Choose one:**   ¾ cup cottage cheese
3 oz. grass-fed beef, chicken breast or pork
Alternate protein: _____
Vegetable = 1-2 servings fresh or frozen – lightly steamed, roasted or baked
Fish Oil capsules = 2 @ 300 mg total combined EPA & DHA (from sardines, anchovies, salmon, mackerel)
1 additional food item allowed:

_____

Meal #4 (3 hours later) **Time:** _____
Water = 16 oz. (must be completely consumed prior to eating)
Protein = 20g **Choose one:** 1cup plain Greek yogurt
6 oz. wild caught fresh fish3 oz. grass-fed beef, chicken breast or pork
1-2 scoop protein powder mixed w/ 20 oz. water
Alternate protein: _____
Nuts = ¼ cup (almonds, brazil, pecans, walnuts) **OR**
Vegetable = 1 serving fresh or frozen – lightly steamed, roasted or baked
NO additional foods consumed

Meal #5 (3 hours later) **Time:** _____
Water = 16 oz. (must be completely consumed prior to eating)
Protein = 20g **Choose one:** 6 oz. wild caught fresh fish
3 oz. grass-fed beef, chicken breast or pork
Alternate protein: _____
Vegetable = 2-3 servings fresh or frozen – lightly steamed, roasted or baked
Fish Oil capsules = 2 @ 300 mg total combined EPA & DHA (from sardines, anchovies, salmon, mackerel)
1 additional food item allowed:
_____

WEEK FIVE: Achieve healthy eating
DAY FOUR: _____

WEEK FIVE INTENTION (Repeat aloud 5 times in the morning and 5 times at night. Repeat silently 3 times prior to each meal):

I SIMPLIFY

Meal #1 (within one hour of awakening) **Time:** _____

Water = 16 oz. (must be completely consumed prior to eating)

Protein = 20g **Choose one:**   1 cup plain Greek yogurt   3 eggs

1-2 scoop protein powder mixed w/ 20 oz. water

Alternate protein: _____

Fruit = small to medium piece _____

Vegetable = 2 T flax, wheat germ, dried greens

Fish Oil capsules = 2 @ 300 mg total combined EPA & DHA (from sardines, anchovies, salmon, mackerel)

Meal #2 (3 hours later) **Time:** _____

Water = 16 oz. (must be completely consumed prior to eating)

Protein = 20g **Choose one:**   ¾ cup cottage cheese   ½ can tuna

Alternate protein: _____

Vegetable = 1 serving fresh or frozen – lightly steamed, roasted or baked

NO additional foods consumed

Meal #3 (3 hours later) **Time:** _____

Water = 16 oz. (must be completely consumed prior to eating)

Protein = 20g **Choose one:**   ¾ cup cottage cheese

3 oz. grass-fed beef, chicken breast or pork

Alternate protein: _____

Vegetable = 1-2 servings fresh or frozen – lightly steamed, roasted or baked

Fish Oil capsules = 2 @ 300 mg total combined EPA & DHA (from sardines, anchovies, salmon, mackerel)

1 additional food item allowed:

_____

Meal #4 (3 hours later) **Time:** _____
Water = 16 oz. (must be completely consumed prior to eating)
Protein = 20g **Choose one:**   1cup plain Greek yogurt
6 oz. wild caught fresh fish3 oz. grass-fed beef, chicken breast or pork
1-2 scoop protein powder mixed w/ 20 oz. water
Alternate protein: _____
Nuts = ¼ cup (almonds, brazil, pecans, walnuts) **OR**
Vegetable = 1 serving fresh or frozen – lightly steamed, roasted or baked
NO additional foods consumed

Meal #5 (3 hours later) **Time:** _____
Water = 16 oz. (must be completely consumed prior to eating)
Protein = 20g **Choose one:**   6 oz. wild caught fresh fish
3 oz. grass-fed beef, chicken breast or pork
Alternate protein: _____
Vegetable = 2-3 servings fresh or frozen – lightly steamed, roasted or baked
Fish Oil capsules = 2 @ 300 mg total combined EPA & DHA (from sardines, anchovies, salmon, mackerel)
1 additional food item allowed:
_____

WEEK FIVE: Achieve healthy eating
DAY FIVE: _____

WEEK FIVE INTENTION (Repeat aloud 5 times in the morning and 5 times at night. Repeat silently 3 times prior to each meal):

I SIMPLIFY

Meal #1 (within one hour of awakening) **Time:** _____
Water = 16 oz. (must be completely consumed prior to eating)
Protein = 20g **Choose one:**　　　1 cup plain Greek yogurt　　　　　3 eggs
1-2 scoop protein powder mixed w/ 20 oz. water
Alternate protein: _____
Fruit = small to medium piece _____
Vegetable = 2 T flax, wheat germ, dried greens
Fish Oil capsules = 2 @ 300 mg total combined EPA & DHA (from sardines, anchovies, salmon, mackerel)

Meal #2 (3 hours later) **Time:** _____
Water = 16 oz. (must be completely consumed prior to eating)
Protein = 20g **Choose one:**　　　¾ cup cottage cheese　　　½ can tuna
Alternate protein: _____
Vegetable = 1 serving fresh or frozen – lightly steamed, roasted or baked
NO additional foods consumed

Meal #3 (3 hours later) **Time:** _____
Water = 16 oz. (must be completely consumed prior to eating)
Protein = 20g **Choose one:**　　　¾ cup cottage cheese
3 oz. grass-fed beef, chicken breast or pork
Alternate protein: _____
Vegetable = 1-2 servings fresh or frozen – lightly steamed, roasted or baked
Fish Oil capsules = 2 @ 300 mg total combined EPA & DHA (from sardines, anchovies, salmon, mackerel)
1 additional food item allowed:

_____

Meal #4 (3 hours later)   Time: _____

Water = 16 oz. (must be completely consumed prior to eating)

Protein = 20g **Choose one:**   1cup plain Greek yogurt

6 oz. wild caught fresh fish3 oz. grass-fed beef, chicken breast or pork

1-2 scoop protein powder mixed w/ 20 oz. water

Alternate protein: _____

Nuts = ¼ cup (almonds, brazil, pecans, walnuts) **OR**

Vegetable = 1 serving fresh or frozen – lightly steamed, roasted or baked

NO additional foods consumed

Meal #5 (3 hours later)   Time: _____

Water = 16 oz. (must be completely consumed prior to eating)

Protein = 20g **Choose one:**   6 oz. wild caught fresh fish

3 oz. grass-fed beef, chicken breast or pork

Alternate protein: _____

Vegetable = 2-3 servings fresh or frozen – lightly steamed, roasted or baked

Fish Oil capsules = 2 @ 300 mg total combined EPA & DHA (from sardines, anchovies, salmon, mackerel)

1 additional food item allowed:

_____

WEEK FIVE: Achieve healthy eating
DAY SIX: _____

WEEK FIVE INTENTION (Repeat aloud 5 times in the morning and 5 times at night. Repeat silently 3 times prior to each meal):

I SIMPLIFY

# Meal #1 (within one hour of awakening) **Time:** _____
Water = 16 oz. (must be completely consumed prior to eating)
Protein = 20g **<u>Choose one:</u>**   1 cup plain Greek yogurt   3 eggs
1-2 scoop protein powder mixed w/ 20 oz. water
Alternate protein: _____
Fruit = small to medium piece _____
Vegetable = 2 T flax, wheat germ, dried greens
Fish Oil capsules = 2 @ 300 mg total combined EPA & DHA (from sardines, anchovies, salmon, mackerel)

# Meal #2 (3 hours later) **Time:** _____
Water = 16 oz. (must be completely consumed prior to eating)
Protein = 20g **<u>Choose one:</u>**   ¾ cup cottage cheese   ½ can tuna
Alternate protein: _____
Vegetable = 1 serving fresh or frozen – lightly steamed, roasted or baked
NO additional foods consumed

# Meal #3 (3 hours later) **Time:** _____
Water = 16 oz. (must be completely consumed prior to eating)
Protein = 20g **<u>Choose one:</u>**   ¾ cup cottage cheese
3 oz. grass-fed beef, chicken breast or pork
Alternate protein: _____
Vegetable = 1-2 servings fresh or frozen – lightly steamed, roasted or baked
Fish Oil capsules = 2 @ 300 mg total combined EPA & DHA (from sardines, anchovies, salmon, mackerel)
1 additional food item allowed:

_____

Meal #4 (3 hours later) **Time:** _____
Water = 16 oz. (must be completely consumed prior to eating)
Protein = 20g **Choose one:**   1cup plain Greek yogurt
6 oz. wild caught fresh fish3 oz. grass-fed beef, chicken breast or pork
1-2 scoop protein powder mixed w/ 20 oz. water
Alternate protein: _____
Nuts = ¼ cup (almonds, brazil, pecans, walnuts) **OR**
Vegetable = 1 serving fresh or frozen – lightly steamed, roasted or baked
NO additional foods consumed

Meal #5 (3 hours later) **Time:** _____
Water = 16 oz. (must be completely consumed prior to eating)
Protein = 20g **Choose one:**   6 oz. wild caught fresh fish
3 oz. grass-fed beef, chicken breast or pork
Alternate protein: _____
Vegetable = 2-3 servings fresh or frozen – lightly steamed, roasted or baked
Fish Oil capsules = 2 @ 300 mg total combined EPA & DHA (from sardines,
anchovies, salmon, mackerel)
1 additional food item allowed:
_____

WEEK FIVE: Achieve healthy eating
DAY SEVEN: _____

WEEK FIVE INTENTION (Repeat aloud 5 times in the morning and 5 times at night. Repeat silently 3 times prior to each meal):

I SIMPLIFY

Meal #1 (within one hour of awakening) **Time:** _____
Water = 16 oz. (must be completely consumed prior to eating)
Protein = 20g <u>**Choose one:**</u>   1 cup plain Greek yogurt   3 eggs
1-2 scoop protein powder mixed w/ 20 oz. water
Alternate protein: _____
Fruit = small to medium piece _____
Vegetable = 2 T flax, wheat germ, dried greens
Fish Oil capsules = 2 @ 300 mg total combined EPA & DHA (from sardines, anchovies, salmon, mackerel)

Meal #2 (3 hours later) **Time:** _____
Water = 16 oz. (must be completely consumed prior to eating)
Protein = 20g <u>**Choose one:**</u>   ¾ cup cottage cheese   ½ can tuna
Alternate protein: _____
Vegetable = 1 serving fresh or frozen – lightly steamed, roasted or baked
NO additional foods consumed

Meal #3 (3 hours later) **Time:** _____
Water = 16 oz. (must be completely consumed prior to eating)
Protein = 20g <u>**Choose one:**</u>   ¾ cup cottage cheese
3 oz. grass-fed beef, chicken breast or pork
Alternate protein: _____
Vegetable = 1-2 servings fresh or frozen – lightly steamed, roasted or baked
Fish Oil capsules = 2 @ 300 mg total combined EPA & DHA (from sardines, anchovies, salmon, mackerel)
1 additional food item allowed:

_____

Meal #4 (3 hours later) **Time:** _____
Water = 16 oz. (must be completely consumed prior to eating)
Protein = 20g **Choose one:**   1cup plain Greek yogurt
6 oz. wild caught fresh fish3 oz. grass-fed beef, chicken breast or pork
1-2 scoop protein powder mixed w/ 20 oz. water
Alternate protein: _____
Nuts = ¼ cup (almonds, brazil, pecans, walnuts) **OR**
Vegetable = 1 serving fresh or frozen – lightly steamed, roasted or baked
NO additional foods consumed

Meal #5 (3 hours later) **Time:** _____
Water = 16 oz. (must be completely consumed prior to eating)
Protein = 20g **Choose one:**   6 oz. wild caught fresh fish
3 oz. grass-fed beef, chicken breast or pork
Alternate protein: _____
Vegetable = 2-3 servings fresh or frozen – lightly steamed, roasted or baked
Fish Oil capsules = 2 @ 300 mg total combined EPA & DHA (from sardines,
anchovies, salmon, mackerel)
1 additional food item allowed:
_____

WEEK SIX: Achieve a healthy metabolism

Week Six may result in big changes in your body composition. At this point, your body has adjusted to the new way of eating and is thriving. Your metabolism is healthier, and you are reaping the benefits. It may be time to consult with your doctor regarding decreasing medications related to obesity and metabolic syndrome.

This week provides you with one meal when you can consume foods that don't contribute to health or lean gains. You may be willing and ready to follow a regimen of healthy food choices and may no longer desire unhealthy foods. You may be motivated by the awesome results you are achieving. Your success is imminent.

To sum up, by the end of Week Six, you will have established:
- A new relationship with food: as fuel and sustenance
- Consistently healthy food choices
- The ability to get right back on Plan should you fall off
- A positive cycle of health and lean results

WEEK SIX: Achieve a healthy metabolism
DAY ONE: _____

WEEK SIX INTENTION (Repeat aloud 5 times in the morning and 5 times at night. Repeat silently 3 times prior to each meal):

I CLOSELY FOLLOW MY PATH TO HEALTH AND WELL BEING

Abdomen msmt: _____   **Waist msmt:** _____   **Hip msmt:** _____

# Meal #1 (within one hour of awakening) **Time:** _____
Water = 16 oz. (must be completely consumed prior to eating)
Protein = 20g **Choose one:**   1 cup plain Greek yogurt   3 eggs
1-2 scoop protein powder mixed w/ 20 oz. water
Alternate protein: _____
Fruit = small to medium piece _____
Vegetable = 2 T flax, wheat germ, dried greens
Fish Oil capsules = 2 @ 300 mg total combined EPA & DHA (from sardines, anchovies, salmon, mackerel)

# Meal #2 (3 hours later) **Time:** _____
Water = 16 oz. (must be completely consumed prior to eating)
Protein = 20g **Choose one:**   ¾ cup cottage cheese   ½ can tuna
Alternate protein: _____
Vegetable = 1 serving fresh or frozen – lightly steamed, roasted or baked

# Meal #3 (3 hours later) **Time:** _____
Water = 16 oz. (must be completely consumed prior to eating)
Protein = 20g **Choose one:**   ¾ cup cottage cheese
3 oz. grass-fed beef, chicken breast or pork
Alternate protein: _____
Vegetable = 1-2 servings fresh or frozen – lightly steamed, roasted or baked
Fish Oil capsules = 2 @ 300 mg total combined EPA & DHA (from sardines, anchovies, salmon, mackerel)
NO additional foods consumed

Meal #4 (3 hours later) **Time:** _____
Water = 16 oz. (must be completely consumed prior to eating)
Protein = 20g **Choose one:**   1cup plain Greek yogurt
6 oz. wild caught fresh fish   3 oz. grass-fed beef, chicken breast or pork
1-2 scoop protein powder mixed w/ 20 oz. water
Alternate protein: _____
Nuts = ¼ cup (almonds, brazil, pecans, walnuts) **OR**
Vegetable = 1 serving fresh or frozen – lightly steamed, roasted or baked

Meal #5 (3 hours later) **Time:** _____
Water = 16 oz. (must be completely consumed prior to eating)
Protein = 20g **Choose one:**   6 oz. wild caught fresh fish
3 oz. grass-fed beef, chicken breast or pork
Alternate protein: _____

Vegetable = 2-3 servings fresh or frozen – lightly steamed, roasted or baked
Fish Oil capsules = 2 @ 300 mg total combined EPA & DHA (from sardines,
anchovies, salmon, mackerel)
1 additional food item allowed:
_____

WEEK SIX: Achieve a healthy metabolism
DAY TWO: _____

WEEK SIX INTENTION (Repeat aloud 5 times in the morning and 5 times at night. Repeat silently 3 times prior to each meal):
I CLOSELY FOLLOW MY PATH TO HEALTH AND WELL BEING

Meal #1 (within one hour of awakening) **Time:** _____
Water = 16 oz. (must be completely consumed prior to eating)
Protein = 20g **Choose one:**   1 cup plain Greek yogurt   3 eggs
1-2 scoop protein powder mixed w/ 20 oz. water
Alternate protein: _____
Fruit = small to medium piece _____
Vegetable = 2 T flax, wheat germ, dried greens
Fish Oil capsules = 2 @ 300 mg total combined EPA & DHA (from sardines, anchovies, salmon, mackerel)

Meal #2 (3 hours later) **Time:** _____
Water = 16 oz. (must be completely consumed prior to eating)
Protein = 20g **Choose one:**   ¾ cup cottage cheese   ½ can tuna
Alternate protein: _____

Vegetable = 1 serving fresh or frozen – lightly steamed, roasted or baked

Meal #3 (3 hours later) **Time:** _____
Water = 16 oz. (must be completely consumed prior to eating)
Protein = 20g **Choose one:**   ¾ cup cottage cheese
3 oz. grass-fed beef, chicken breast or pork
Alternate protein: _____

Vegetable = 1-2 servings fresh or frozen – lightly steamed, roasted or baked
Fish Oil capsules = 2 @ 300 mg total combined EPA & DHA (from sardines, anchovies, salmon, mackerel)
NO additional foods consumed

Meal #4 (3 hours later) **Time:** _____

Water = 16 oz. (must be completely consumed prior to eating)

Protein = 20g **Choose one:**　　　1 cup plain Greek yogurt

6 oz. wild caught fresh fish　　　3 oz. grass-fed beef, chicken breast or pork

1-2 scoop protein powder mixed w/ 20 oz. water

Alternate protein: _____

Nuts = ¼ cup (almonds, brazil, pecans, walnuts) **OR**

Vegetable = 1 serving fresh or frozen – lightly steamed, roasted or baked

Meal #5 (3 hours later) **Time:** _____

Water = 16 oz. (must be completely consumed prior to eating)

Protein = 20g **Choose one:**　　　6 oz. wild caught fresh fish

3 oz. grass-fed beef, chicken breast or pork

Alternate protein: _____

Vegetable = 2-3 servings fresh or frozen – lightly steamed, roasted or baked

Fish Oil capsules = 2 @ 300 mg total combined EPA & DHA (from sardines, anchovies, salmon, mackerel)

1 additional food item allowed:

WEEK SIX: Achieve a healthy metabolism
DAY THREE: _____

WEEK SIX INTENTION (Repeat aloud 5 times in the morning and 5 times at night. Repeat silently 3 times prior to each meal):
I CLOSELY FOLLOW MY PATH TO HEALTH AND WELL BEING

# Meal #1 (within one hour of awakening) **Time:** _____
Water = 16 oz. (must be completely consumed prior to eating)
Protein = 20g **Choose one:**   1 cup plain Greek yogurt   3 eggs
1-2 scoop protein powder mixed w/ 20 oz. water
Alternate protein: _____
Fruit = small to medium piece _____
Vegetable = 2 T flax, wheat germ, dried greens
Fish Oil capsules = 2 @ 300 mg total combined EPA & DHA (from sardines, anchovies, salmon, mackerel)

# Meal #2 (3 hours later) **Time:** _____
Water = 16 oz. (must be completely consumed prior to eating)
Protein = 20g **Choose one:**   ¾ cup cottage cheese   ½ can tuna
Alternate protein: _____

Vegetable = 1 serving fresh or frozen – lightly steamed, roasted or baked

# Meal #3 (3 hours later) **Time:** _____
Water = 16 oz. (must be completely consumed prior to eating)
Protein = 20g **Choose one:**   ¾ cup cottage cheese
3 oz. grass-fed beef, chicken breast or pork
Alternate protein: _____

Vegetable = 1-2 servings fresh or frozen – lightly steamed, roasted or baked
Fish Oil capsules = 2 @ 300 mg total combined EPA & DHA (from sardines, anchovies, salmon, mackerel)
NO additional foods consumed

Meal #4 (3 hours later)   **Time:** _____

Water = 16 oz. (must be completely consumed prior to eating)

Protein = 20g **Choose one:**   1cup plain Greek yogurt

6 oz. wild caught fresh fish   3 oz. grass-fed beef, chicken breast or pork

1-2 scoop protein powder mixed w/ 20 oz. water

Alternate protein: _____

Nuts = ¼ cup (almonds, brazil, pecans, walnuts) **OR**

Vegetable = 1 serving fresh or frozen – lightly steamed, roasted or baked

Meal #5 (3 hours later)   **Time:** _____

Water = 16 oz. (must be completely consumed prior to eating)

Protein = 20g **Choose one:**   6 oz. wild caught fresh fish

3 oz. grass-fed beef, chicken breast or pork

Alternate protein: _____

Vegetable = 2-3 servings fresh or frozen – lightly steamed, roasted or baked

Fish Oil capsules = 2 @ 300 mg total combined EPA & DHA (from sardines, anchovies, salmon, mackerel)

1 additional food item allowed:

_____

WEEK SIX: Achieve a healthy metabolism
DAY FOUR: _____

WEEK SIX INTENTION (Repeat aloud 5 times in the morning and 5 times at night. Repeat silently 3 times prior to each meal):
I CLOSELY FOLLOW MY PATH TO HEALTH AND WELL BEING

Meal #1 (within one hour of awakening) **Time:** _____
Water = 16 oz. (must be completely consumed prior to eating)
Protein = 20g **Choose one:**   1 cup plain Greek yogurt   3 eggs
1-2 scoop protein powder mixed w/ 20 oz. water
Alternate protein: _____
Fruit = small to medium piece _____
Vegetable = 2 T flax, wheat germ, dried greens
Fish Oil capsules = 2 @ 300 mg total combined EPA & DHA (from sardines, anchovies, salmon, mackerel)

Meal #2 (3 hours later) **Time:** _____
Water = 16 oz. (must be completely consumed prior to eating)
Protein = 20g **Choose one:**   ¾ cup cottage cheese   ½ can tuna
Alternate protein: _____
Vegetable = 1 serving fresh or frozen – lightly steamed, roasted or baked

Meal #3 (3 hours later) **Time:** _____
Water = 16 oz. (must be completely consumed prior to eating)
Protein = 20g **Choose one:**   ¾ cup cottage cheese
3 oz. grass-fed beef, chicken breast or pork
Alternate protein: _____
Vegetable = 1-2 servings fresh or frozen – lightly steamed, roasted or baked
Fish Oil capsules = 2 @ 300 mg total combined EPA & DHA (from sardines, anchovies, salmon, mackerel)
NO additional foods consumed

Meal #4 (3 hours later) **Time:** _____

Water = 16 oz. (must be completely consumed prior to eating)

Protein = 20g **Choose one:**   1cup plain Greek yogurt

6 oz. wild caught fresh fish   3 oz. grass-fed beef, chicken breast or pork

1-2 scoop protein powder mixed w/ 20 oz. water

Alternate protein: _____

Nuts = ¼ cup (almonds, brazil, pecans, walnuts) **OR**

Vegetable = 1 serving fresh or frozen – lightly steamed, roasted or baked

Meal #5 (3 hours later) **Time:** _____

Water = 16 oz. (must be completely consumed prior to eating)

Protein = 20g **Choose one:**   6 oz. wild caught fresh fish

3 oz. grass-fed beef, chicken breast or pork

Alternate protein: _____

Vegetable = 2-3 servings fresh or frozen – lightly steamed, roasted or baked

Fish Oil capsules = 2 @ 300 mg total combined EPA & DHA (from sardines, anchovies, salmon, mackerel)

1 additional food item allowed:

WEEK SIX: Achieve a healthy metabolism
DAY FIVE: _____

WEEK SIX INTENTION (Repeat aloud 5 times in the morning and 5 times at night. Repeat silently 3 times prior to each meal):
I CLOSELY FOLLOW MY PATH TO HEALTH AND WELL BEING

Meal #1 (within one hour of awakening) **Time:** _____
Water = 16 oz. (must be completely consumed prior to eating)
Protein = 20g **Choose one:**   1 cup plain Greek yogurt   3 eggs
1-2 scoop protein powder mixed w/ 20 oz. water
Alternate protein: _____
Fruit = small to medium piece _____
Vegetable = 2 T flax, wheat germ, dried greens
Fish Oil capsules = 2 @ 300 mg total combined EPA & DHA (from sardines, anchovies, salmon, mackerel)

Meal #2 (3 hours later) **Time:** _____
Water = 16 oz. (must be completely consumed prior to eating)
Protein = 20g **Choose one:**   ¾ cup cottage cheese   ½ can tuna
Alternate protein: _____

Vegetable = 1 serving fresh or frozen – lightly steamed, roasted or baked

Meal #3 (3 hours later) **Time:** _____
Water = 16 oz. (must be completely consumed prior to eating)
Protein = 20g **Choose one:**   ¾ cup cottage cheese
3 oz. grass-fed beef, chicken breast or pork
Alternate protein: _____

Vegetable = 1-2 servings fresh or frozen – lightly steamed, roasted or baked
Fish Oil capsules = 2 @ 300 mg total combined EPA & DHA (from sardines, anchovies, salmon, mackerel)
NO additional foods consumed

Meal #4 (3 hours later) **Time:** _____

Water = 16 oz. (must be completely consumed prior to eating)

Protein = 20g **Choose one:**   1cup plain Greek yogurt

6 oz. wild caught fresh fish   3 oz. grass-fed beef, chicken breast or pork

1-2 scoop protein powder mixed w/ 20 oz. water

Alternate protein: _____

Nuts = ¼ cup (almonds, brazil, pecans, walnuts) **OR**

Vegetable = 1 serving fresh or frozen – lightly steamed, roasted or baked

Meal #5 (3 hours later) **Time:** _____

Water = 16 oz. (must be completely consumed prior to eating)

Protein = 20g **Choose one:**   6 oz. wild caught fresh fish

3 oz. grass-fed beef, chicken breast or pork

Alternate protein: _____

Vegetable = 2-3 servings fresh or frozen – lightly steamed, roasted or baked

Fish Oil capsules = 2 @ 300 mg total combined EPA & DHA (from sardines, anchovies, salmon, mackerel)

1 additional food item allowed:

_____

WEEK SIX: Achieve a healthy metabolism
DAY SIX: _____

WEEK SIX INTENTION (Repeat aloud 5 times in the morning and 5 times at night. Repeat silently 3 times prior to each meal):
I CLOSELY FOLLOW MY PATH TO HEALTH AND WELL BEING

# Meal #1 (within one hour of awakening) **Time:** _____
Water = 16 oz. (must be completely consumed prior to eating)
Protein = 20g **Choose one:**   1 cup plain Greek yogurt   3 eggs
1-2 scoop protein powder mixed w/ 20 oz. water
Alternate protein: _____
Fruit = small to medium piece _____
Vegetable = 2 T flax, wheat germ, dried greens
Fish Oil capsules = 2 @ 300 mg total combined EPA & DHA (from sardines, anchovies, salmon, mackerel)

# Meal #2 (3 hours later) **Time:** _____
Water = 16 oz. (must be completely consumed prior to eating)
Protein = 20g **Choose one:**   ¾ cup cottage cheese   ½ can tuna
Alternate protein: _____

Vegetable = 1 serving fresh or frozen – lightly steamed, roasted or baked

# Meal #3 (3 hours later) **Time:** _____
Water = 16 oz. (must be completely consumed prior to eating)
Protein = 20g **Choose one:**   ¾ cup cottage cheese
3 oz. grass-fed beef, chicken breast or pork
Alternate protein: _____

Vegetable = 1-2 servings fresh or frozen – lightly steamed, roasted or baked
Fish Oil capsules = 2 @ 300 mg total combined EPA & DHA (from sardines, anchovies, salmon, mackerel)
NO additional foods consumed

Meal #4 (3 hours later) **Time:** _____
Water = 16 oz. (must be completely consumed prior to eating)
Protein = 20g **Choose one:**   1cup plain Greek yogurt
6 oz. wild caught fresh fish   3 oz. grass-fed beef, chicken breast or pork
1-2 scoop protein powder mixed w/ 20 oz. water
Alternate protein: _____
Nuts = ¼ cup (almonds, brazil, pecans, walnuts) **OR**
Vegetable = 1 serving fresh or frozen – lightly steamed, roasted or baked

Meal #5 (3 hours later) **Time:** _____
Water = 16 oz. (must be completely consumed prior to eating)
Protein = 20g **Choose one:**   6 oz. wild caught fresh fish
3 oz. grass-fed beef, chicken breast or pork
Alternate protein: _____

Vegetable = 2-3 servings fresh or frozen – lightly steamed, roasted or baked
Fish Oil capsules = 2 @ 300 mg total combined EPA & DHA (from sardines, anchovies, salmon, mackerel)
1 additional food item allowed:

WEEK SIX: Achieve a healthy metabolism
DAY SEVEN: _____

WEEK SIX INTENTION (Repeat aloud 5 times in the morning and 5 times at night. Repeat silently 3 times prior to each meal):

I CLOSELY FOLLOW MY PATH TO HEALTH AND WELL BEING

Meal #1 (within one hour of awakening) **Time:** _____
Water = 16 oz. (must be completely consumed prior to eating)
Protein = 20g **Choose one:**   1 cup plain Greek yogurt   3 eggs
1-2 scoop protein powder mixed w/ 20 oz. water
Alternate protein: _____
Fruit = small to medium piece _____
Vegetable = 2 T flax, wheat germ, dried greens
Fish Oil capsules = 2 @ 300 mg total combined EPA & DHA (from sardines, anchovies, salmon, mackerel)

Meal #2 (3 hours later) **Time:** _____
Water = 16 oz. (must be completely consumed prior to eating)
Protein = 20g **Choose one:**   ¾ cup cottage cheese   ½ can tuna
Alternate protein: _____

Vegetable = 1 serving fresh or frozen – lightly steamed, roasted or baked

Meal #3 (3 hours later) **Time:** _____
Water = 16 oz. (must be completely consumed prior to eating)
Protein = 20g **Choose one:**   ¾ cup cottage cheese
3 oz. grass-fed beef, chicken breast or pork
Alternate protein: _____

Vegetable = 1-2 servings fresh or frozen – lightly steamed, roasted or baked
Fish Oil capsules = 2 @ 300 mg total combined EPA & DHA (from sardines, anchovies, salmon, mackerel)
NO additional foods consumed

Meal #4 (3 hours later) **Time:** _____

Water = 16 oz. (must be completely consumed prior to eating)

Protein = 20g **Choose one:**   1cup plain Greek yogurt

6 oz. wild caught fresh fish   3 oz. grass-fed beef, chicken breast or pork

1-2 scoop protein powder mixed w/ 20 oz. water

Alternate protein: _____

Nuts = ¼ cup (almonds, brazil, pecans, walnuts) **OR**

Vegetable = 1 serving fresh or frozen – lightly steamed, roasted or baked

Meal #5 (3 hours later) **Time:** _____

Water = 16 oz. (must be completely consumed prior to eating)

Protein = 20g **Choose one:**   6 oz. wild caught fresh fish

3 oz. grass-fed beef, chicken breast or pork

Alternate protein: _____

Vegetable = 2-3 servings fresh or frozen – lightly steamed, roasted or baked

Fish Oil capsules = 2 @ 300 mg total combined EPA & DHA (from sardines, anchovies, salmon, mackerel)

1 additional food item allowed:

_____

WEEK SEVEN: Achieve wellness

Week Seven is a continuation of Week Six as you continue becoming healthy, strong, functional and lean. You are now well aware of your food choices and are more educated regarding healthy versus unhealthy foods. You have established the baseline of systematic eating, consuming adequate water, protein and fiber-rich foods.

We add a bit more carbohydrate into the Plan in the first meal in the form of oatmeal or whole grain bread. The fruit is optional at this point. You still have the freedom to include less healthy foods in the final meal of the day, but you will probably be avoiding the unhealthy choices on most days.

To sum up, by the end of Week Seven, you will have established:
- Health and wellness
- Optimal strength and functional movement
- A lean physique

WEEK SEVEN: Achieve wellness
DAY ONE: _____

WEEK SEVEN INTENTION (Repeat aloud 5 times in the morning and 5 times at night. Repeat silently 3 times prior to each meal):
I AM SUCCESSFUL

Abdomen msmt: _____   **Waist msmt:** _____   **Hip msmt:** _____

Meal #1 (within one hour of awakening) Time: _____
Water = 16 oz. (must be completely consumed prior to eating)
Protein = ___ g: _____
Fruit = small to medium piece
Carbohydrate = 1 cup non-instant oatmeal OR slice whole grain bread
Vegetable = 2 T flax, wheat germ, dried greens
Fish Oil capsules = 2 @ 300 mg total combined EPA & DHA (from sardines, anchovies, salmon, mackerel)

Meal #2 (3 hours later) Time: _____
Water = 16 oz. (must be completely consumed prior to eating)
Protein = ___ g: _____
Vegetable = 1 serving fresh or frozen – lightly steamed, roasted or baked

Meal #3 (3 hours later) Time: _____
Water = 16 oz. (must be completely consumed prior to eating)
Protein = ___ g: _____
Vegetable = 1-2 servings fresh or frozen – lightly steamed, roasted or baked
Fish Oil capsules = 2 @ 300 mg total combined EPA & DHA (from sardines, anchovies, salmon, mackerel)

Meal #4 (3 hours later) Time: _____
Water = 16 oz. (must be completely consumed prior to eating)
Protein = ___ g: _____
Nuts = ¼ cup OR Vegetable = 1 serving fresh or frozen – lightly steamed, roasted or baked

Meal #5 (3 hours later) Time: _____
Water = 16 oz. (must be completely consumed prior to eating)
Protein = ___ g: _____
Vegetable = 2-3 servings fresh or frozen – lightly steamed, roasted or baked
1 additional food item allowed:
_____

WEEK SEVEN: Achieve wellness
DAY TWO: _____

WEEK SEVEN INTENTION (Repeat aloud 5 times in the morning and 5 times at night. Repeat silently 3 times prior to each meal):

I AM SUCCESSFUL

Meal #1 (within one hour of awakening) Time: _____
Water = 16 oz. (must be completely consumed prior to eating)
Protein = ___ g: _____
Fruit = small to medium piece
Carbohydrate = 1 cup non-instant oatmeal OR slice whole grain bread
Vegetable = 2 T flax, wheat germ, dried greens
Fish Oil capsules = 2 @ 300 mg total combined EPA & DHA (from sardines, anchovies, salmon, mackerel)

Meal #2 (3 hours later) Time: _____
Water = 16 oz. (must be completely consumed prior to eating)
Protein = ___ g: _____
Vegetable = 1 serving fresh or frozen – lightly steamed, roasted or baked

Meal #3 (3 hours later) Time: _____
Water = 16 oz. (must be completely consumed prior to eating)
Protein = ___ g: _____
Vegetable = 1-2 servings fresh or frozen – lightly steamed, roasted or baked
Fish Oil capsules = 2 @ 300 mg total combined EPA & DHA (from sardines, anchovies, salmon, mackerel)

Meal #4 (3 hours later) Time: _____

Water = 16 oz. (must be completely consumed prior to eating)

Protein = ___ g: _____

Nuts = ¼ cup OR Vegetable = 1 serving fresh or frozen – lightly steamed, roasted or baked

Meal #5 (3 hours later) Time: _____

Water = 16 oz. (must be completely consumed prior to eating)

Protein = ___ g: _____

Vegetable = 2-3 servings fresh or frozen – lightly steamed, roasted or baked

1 additional food item allowed:

_____

WEEK SEVEN: Achieve wellness
DAY THREE: _____

WEEK SEVEN INTENTION (Repeat aloud 5 times in the morning and 5 times at night. Repeat silently 3 times prior to each meal):

I AM SUCCESSFUL

Meal #1 (within one hour of awakening) Time: _____
Water = 16 oz. (must be completely consumed prior to eating)
Protein = ___ g: _____
Fruit = small to medium piece
Carbohydrate = 1 cup non-instant oatmeal OR slice whole grain bread
Vegetable = 2 T flax, wheat germ, dried greens
Fish Oil capsules = 2 @ 300 mg total combined EPA & DHA (from sardines, anchovies, salmon, mackerel)

Meal #2 (3 hours later) Time: _____
Water = 16 oz. (must be completely consumed prior to eating)
Protein = ___ g: _____
Vegetable = 1 serving fresh or frozen – lightly steamed, roasted or baked

Meal #3 (3 hours later) Time: _____
Water = 16 oz. (must be completely consumed prior to eating)
Protein = ___ g: _____
Vegetable = 1-2 servings fresh or frozen – lightly steamed, roasted or baked
Fish Oil capsules = 2 @ 300 mg total combined EPA & DHA (from sardines, anchovies, salmon, mackerel)

Meal #4 (3 hours later) Time: _____

Water = 16 oz. (must be completely consumed prior to eating)

Protein = ___ g: _____

Nuts = ¼ cup OR Vegetable = 1 serving fresh or frozen – lightly steamed, roasted or baked

Meal #5 (3 hours later) Time: _____

Water = 16 oz. (must be completely consumed prior to eating)

Protein = ___ g: _____

Vegetable = 2-3 servings fresh or frozen – lightly steamed, roasted or baked

1 additional food item allowed:

_____

WEEK SEVEN: Achieve wellness
DAY FOUR: _____

WEEK SEVEN INTENTION (Repeat aloud 5 times in the morning and 5 times at night. Repeat silently 3 times prior to each meal):

I AM SUCCESSFUL

Meal #1 (within one hour of awakening) Time: _____
Water = 16 oz. (must be completely consumed prior to eating)
Protein = ___ g: _____
Fruit = small to medium piece
Carbohydrate = 1 cup non-instant oatmeal OR slice whole grain bread
Vegetable = 2 T flax, wheat germ, dried greens
Fish Oil capsules = 2 @ 300 mg total combined EPA & DHA (from sardines, anchovies, salmon, mackerel)

Meal #2 (3 hours later) Time: _____
Water = 16 oz. (must be completely consumed prior to eating)
Protein = ___ g: _____
Vegetable = 1 serving fresh or frozen – lightly steamed, roasted or baked

Meal #3 (3 hours later) Time: _____
Water = 16 oz. (must be completely consumed prior to eating)
Protein = ___ g: _____
Vegetable = 1-2 servings fresh or frozen – lightly steamed, roasted or baked
Fish Oil capsules = 2 @ 300 mg total combined EPA & DHA (from sardines, anchovies, salmon, mackerel)

Meal #4 (3 hours later) Time: _____

Water = 16 oz. (must be completely consumed prior to eating)

Protein = ___ g: _____

Nuts = ¼ cup OR Vegetable = 1 serving fresh or frozen – lightly steamed, roasted or baked

Meal #5 (3 hours later) Time: _____

Water = 16 oz. (must be completely consumed prior to eating)

Protein = ___ g: _____

Vegetable = 2-3 servings fresh or frozen – lightly steamed, roasted or baked

1 additional food item allowed:

_____

WEEK SEVEN: Achieve wellness
DAY FIVE: _____

WEEK SEVEN INTENTION (Repeat aloud 5 times in the morning and 5 times at
night. Repeat silently 3 times prior to each meal):
I AM SUCCESSFUL

Meal #1 (within one hour of awakening) Time: _____
Water = 16 oz. (must be completely consumed prior to eating)
Protein = ___ g: _____
Fruit = small to medium piece
Carbohydrate = 1 cup non-instant oatmeal OR slice whole grain bread
Vegetable = 2 T flax, wheat germ, dried greens
Fish Oil capsules = 2 @ 300 mg total combined EPA & DHA (from sardines,
anchovies, salmon, mackerel)

Meal #2 (3 hours later) Time: _____
Water = 16 oz. (must be completely consumed prior to eating)
Protein = ___ g: _____
Vegetable = 1 serving fresh or frozen – lightly steamed, roasted or baked

Meal #3 (3 hours later) Time: _____
Water = 16 oz. (must be completely consumed prior to eating)
Protein = ___ g: _____
Vegetable = 1-2 servings fresh or frozen – lightly steamed, roasted or baked
Fish Oil capsules = 2 @ 300 mg total combined EPA & DHA (from sardines,
anchovies, salmon, mackerel)

Meal #4 (3 hours later) Time: _____

Water = 16 oz. (must be completely consumed prior to eating)

Protein = ___ g: _____

Nuts = ¼ cup OR Vegetable = 1 serving fresh or frozen – lightly steamed, roasted or baked

Meal #5 (3 hours later) Time: _____

Water = 16 oz. (must be completely consumed prior to eating)

Protein = ___ g: _____

Vegetable = 2-3 servings fresh or frozen – lightly steamed, roasted or baked

1 additional food item allowed:

_____

WEEK SEVEN: Achieve wellness
DAY SIX: _____

WEEK SEVEN INTENTION (Repeat aloud 5 times in the morning and 5 times at night. Repeat silently 3 times prior to each meal):

I AM SUCCESSFUL

Meal #1 (within one hour of awakening) Time: _____
Water = 16 oz. (must be completely consumed prior to eating)
Protein = ___ g: _____
Fruit = small to medium piece
Carbohydrate = 1 cup non-instant oatmeal OR slice whole grain bread
Vegetable = 2 T flax, wheat germ, dried greens
Fish Oil capsules = 2 @ 300 mg total combined EPA & DHA (from sardines, anchovies, salmon, mackerel)

Meal #2 (3 hours later) Time: _____
Water = 16 oz. (must be completely consumed prior to eating)
Protein = ___ g: _____
Vegetable = 1 serving fresh or frozen – lightly steamed, roasted or baked

Meal #3 (3 hours later) Time: _____
Water = 16 oz. (must be completely consumed prior to eating)
Protein = ___ g: _____
Vegetable = 1-2 servings fresh or frozen – lightly steamed, roasted or baked
Fish Oil capsules = 2 @ 300 mg total combined EPA & DHA (from sardines, anchovies, salmon, mackerel)

Meal #4 (3 hours later) Time: _____
Water = 16 oz. (must be completely consumed prior to eating)
Protein = ___ g: _____
Nuts = ¼ cup OR Vegetable = 1 serving fresh or frozen – lightly steamed, roasted or baked

Meal #5 (3 hours later) Time: _____
Water = 16 oz. (must be completely consumed prior to eating)
Protein = ___ g: _____
Vegetable = 2-3 servings fresh or frozen – lightly steamed, roasted or baked
1 additional food item allowed:

_____

WEEK SEVEN: Achieve wellness
DAY SEVEN: _____

WEEK SEVEN INTENTION (Repeat aloud 5 times in the morning and 5 times at night. Repeat silently 3 times prior to each meal):

I AM SUCCESSFUL

Meal #1 (within one hour of awakening) Time: _____
Water = 16 oz. (must be completely consumed prior to eating)
Protein = ___ g: _____
Fruit = small to medium piece
Carbohydrate = 1 cup non-instant oatmeal OR slice whole grain bread
Vegetable = 2 T flax, wheat germ, dried greens
Fish Oil capsules = 2 @ 300 mg total combined EPA & DHA (from sardines, anchovies, salmon, mackerel)

Meal #2 (3 hours later) Time: _____
Water = 16 oz. (must be completely consumed prior to eating)
Protein = ___ g: _____
Vegetable = 1 serving fresh or frozen – lightly steamed, roasted or baked

Meal #3 (3 hours later) Time: _____
Water = 16 oz. (must be completely consumed prior to eating)
Protein = ___ g: _____
Vegetable = 1-2 servings fresh or frozen – lightly steamed, roasted or baked
Fish Oil capsules = 2 @ 300 mg total combined EPA & DHA (from sardines, anchovies, salmon, mackerel)

Meal #4 (3 hours later) Time: _____

Water = 16 oz. (must be completely consumed prior to eating)

Protein = ___ g: _____

Nuts = ¼ cup OR Vegetable = 1 serving fresh or frozen – lightly steamed, roasted or baked

Meal #5 (3 hours later) Time: _____

Water = 16 oz. (must be completely consumed prior to eating)

Protein = ___ g: _____

Vegetable = 2-3 servings fresh or frozen – lightly steamed, roasted or baked

1 additional food item allowed:

_____

WEEK EIGHT: Achieve lean!

Congratulations! You have established a strong baseline of healthy food choices and have spent seven weeks rebooting your metabolism so that you are healthy and well. Your body is responding to your exercise protocols and you are making great progress. You can continue beyond Week 8 following that eating plan. Or you can begin to experiment with frequency of eating and food quality. Many individuals do quite well with three meals per day. If you exercise a lot, you may find you want to eat six or seven meals per day.

If you like food choices such as processed foods or alcoholic beverages, you now know that they are not a part of an optimally healthy eating plan. However, if you desire, you can begin to introduce these and other food choices slowly and carefully to determine if they make an impact on your health and lean gains. You will find that you have plenty of flexibility in your eating choices because you have established a healthy metabolism and healthy eating habits. Should you find that your body composition is changing unfavorably, revert back to Week 8 and follow it carefully for a week or two. That should put you right back on track.

Remember to always follow the baseline of the Plan:
- Eat first thing in the morning; eat systematically; consume adequate water, animal proteins and fiber–rich foods.
- Expand the intention recitations with a daily meditation practice.
- Stay active and exercise.

You should feel very proud of yourself. You have created a new relationship with food and have established healthy eating habits that will take you through a lifetime. You have certainly Achieved Lean!

WEEK EIGHT: Achieve lean!
DAY ONE: _____

WEEK EIGHT INTENTION (Repeat aloud 5 times in the morning and 5 times at night. Repeat silently 3 times prior to each meal):

I AM STRONG AND LEAN

Abdomen msmt: _____   **Waist msmt:** _____   **Hip msmt:** _____

# Meal #1 (within one hour of awakening) Time: _____
Water = 16 oz. (must be completely consumed prior to eating)
Protein = ___ g: _____
Fruit = small to medium piece
Carbohydrate = 1 cup non-instant oatmeal OR slice whole grain bread
Vegetable = 2 T flax, wheat germ, dried greens
Fish Oil capsules = 2 @ 300 mg total combined EPA & DHA (from sardines, anchovies, salmon, mackerel)

# Meal #2 (3 hours later) Time: _____
Water = 16 oz. (must be completely consumed prior to eating)
Protein = ___ g: _____
Vegetable = 1 serving fresh or frozen – lightly steamed, roasted or baked

# Meal #3 (3 hours later) Time: _____
Water = 16 oz. (must be completely consumed prior to eating)
Protein = ___ g: _____
Vegetable = 1-2 servings fresh or frozen – lightly steamed, roasted or baked
Fish Oil capsules = 2 @ 300 mg total combined EPA & DHA (from sardines, anchovies, salmon, mackerel)

Meal #4 (3 hours later) Time: _____

Water = 16 oz. (must be completely consumed prior to eating)

Protein = ___ g: _____

Nuts = ¼ cup OR Vegetable = 1 serving fresh or frozen – lightly steamed, roasted or baked

Meal #5 (3 hours later) Time: _____

Water = 16 oz. (must be completely consumed prior to eating)

Protein = ___ g: _____

Vegetable = 2-3 servings fresh or frozen – lightly steamed, roasted or baked

NO additional foods consumed

WEEK EIGHT: Achieve lean!
DAY TWO: _____

WEEK EIGHT INTENTION (Repeat aloud 5 times in the morning and 5 times at night. Repeat silently 3 times prior to each meal):

I AM STRONG AND LEAN

Meal #1 (within one hour of awakening) Time: _____
Water = 16 oz. (must be completely consumed prior to eating)
Protein = ___ g: _____
Fruit = small to medium piece
Carbohydrate = 1 cup non-instant oatmeal OR slice whole grain bread
Vegetable = 2 T flax, wheat germ, dried greens
Fish Oil capsules = 2 @ 300 mg total combined EPA & DHA (from sardines, anchovies, salmon, mackerel)

Meal #2 (3 hours later) Time: _____
Water = 16 oz. (must be completely consumed prior to eating)
Protein = ___ g: _____
Vegetable = 1 serving fresh or frozen – lightly steamed, roasted or baked

Meal #3 (3 hours later) Time: _____
Water = 16 oz. (must be completely consumed prior to eating)
Protein = ___ g: _____
Vegetable = 1-2 servings fresh or frozen – lightly steamed, roasted or baked
Fish Oil capsules = 2 @ 300 mg total combined EPA & DHA (from sardines, anchovies, salmon, mackerel)

Meal #4 (3 hours later) Time: _____

Water = 16 oz. (must be completely consumed prior to eating)

Protein = ___ g: _____

Nuts = ¼ cup OR Vegetable = 1 serving fresh or frozen – lightly steamed, roasted or baked

Meal #5 (3 hours later) Time: _____

Water = 16 oz. (must be completely consumed prior to eating)

Protein = ___ g: _____

Vegetable = 2-3 servings fresh or frozen – lightly steamed, roasted or baked

NO additional foods consumed

WEEK EIGHT: Achieve lean!
DAY THREE: _____

WEEK EIGHT INTENTION (Repeat aloud 5 times in the morning and 5 times at night. Repeat silently 3 times prior to each meal):
I AM STRONG AND LEAN

Meal #1 (within one hour of awakening) Time: _____
Water = 16 oz. (must be completely consumed prior to eating)
Protein = ___ g: _____
Fruit = small to medium piece
Carbohydrate = 1 cup non-instant oatmeal OR slice whole grain bread
Vegetable = 2 T flax, wheat germ, dried greens
Fish Oil capsules = 2 @ 300 mg total combined EPA & DHA (from sardines, anchovies, salmon, mackerel)

Meal #2 (3 hours later) Time: _____
Water = 16 oz. (must be completely consumed prior to eating)
Protein = ___ g: _____
Vegetable = 1 serving fresh or frozen – lightly steamed, roasted or baked

Meal #3 (3 hours later) Time: _____
Water = 16 oz. (must be completely consumed prior to eating)
Protein = ___ g: _____
Vegetable = 1-2 servings fresh or frozen – lightly steamed, roasted or baked
Fish Oil capsules = 2 @ 300 mg total combined EPA & DHA (from sardines, anchovies, salmon, mackerel)

Meal #4 (3 hours later) Time: _____

Water = 16 oz. (must be completely consumed prior to eating)

Protein = ____ g: _____

Nuts = ¼ cup OR Vegetable = 1 serving fresh or frozen – lightly steamed, roasted or baked

Meal #5 (3 hours later) Time: _____

Water = 16 oz. (must be completely consumed prior to eating)

Protein = ____ g: _____

Vegetable = 2-3 servings fresh or frozen – lightly steamed, roasted or baked

NO additional foods consumed

WEEK EIGHT: Achieve lean!
DAY FOUR: _____

WEEK EIGHT INTENTION (Repeat aloud 5 times in the morning and 5 times at night. Repeat silently 3 times prior to each meal):

I AM STRONG AND LEAN

Meal #1 (within one hour of awakening) Time: _____
Water = 16 oz. (must be completely consumed prior to eating)
Protein = ___ g: _____
Fruit = small to medium piece
Carbohydrate = 1 cup non-instant oatmeal OR slice whole grain bread
Vegetable = 2 T flax, wheat germ, dried greens
Fish Oil capsules = 2 @ 300 mg total combined EPA & DHA (from sardines, anchovies, salmon, mackerel)

Meal #2 (3 hours later) Time: _____
Water = 16 oz. (must be completely consumed prior to eating)
Protein = ___ g: _____
Vegetable = 1 serving fresh or frozen – lightly steamed, roasted or baked

Meal #3 (3 hours later) Time: _____
Water = 16 oz. (must be completely consumed prior to eating)
Protein = ___ g: _____
Vegetable = 1-2 servings fresh or frozen – lightly steamed, roasted or baked
Fish Oil capsules = 2 @ 300 mg total combined EPA & DHA (from sardines, anchovies, salmon, mackerel)

Meal #4 (3 hours later) Time: _____

Water = 16 oz. (must be completely consumed prior to eating)

Protein = ___ g: _____

Nuts = ¼ cup OR Vegetable = 1 serving fresh or frozen – lightly steamed, roasted or baked

Meal #5 (3 hours later) Time: _____

Water = 16 oz. (must be completely consumed prior to eating)

Protein = ___ g: _____

Vegetable = 2-3 servings fresh or frozen – lightly steamed, roasted or baked

NO additional foods consumed

WEEK EIGHT: Achieve lean!
DAY FIVE: _____

WEEK EIGHT INTENTION (Repeat aloud 5 times in the morning and 5 times at night. Repeat silently 3 times prior to each meal):

I AM STRONG AND LEAN

Meal #1 (within one hour of awakening) Time: _____
Water = 16 oz. (must be completely consumed prior to eating)
Protein = ___ g: _____
Fruit = small to medium piece
Carbohydrate = 1 cup non-instant oatmeal OR slice whole grain bread
Vegetable = 2 T flax, wheat germ, dried greens
Fish Oil capsules = 2 @ 300 mg total combined EPA & DHA (from sardines, anchovies, salmon, mackerel)

Meal #2 (3 hours later) Time: _____
Water = 16 oz. (must be completely consumed prior to eating)
Protein = ___ g: _____
Vegetable = 1 serving fresh or frozen – lightly steamed, roasted or baked

Meal #3 (3 hours later) Time: _____
Water = 16 oz. (must be completely consumed prior to eating)
Protein = ___ g: _____
Vegetable = 1-2 servings fresh or frozen – lightly steamed, roasted or baked
Fish Oil capsules = 2 @ 300 mg total combined EPA & DHA (from sardines, anchovies, salmon, mackerel)

Meal #4 (3 hours later) Time: _____

Water = 16 oz. (must be completely consumed prior to eating)

Protein = ___ g: _____

Nuts = ¼ cup OR Vegetable = 1 serving fresh or frozen – lightly steamed, roasted or baked

Meal #5 (3 hours later) Time: _____

Water = 16 oz. (must be completely consumed prior to eating)

Protein = ___ g: _____

Vegetable = 2-3 servings fresh or frozen – lightly steamed, roasted or baked

NO additional foods consumed

WEEK EIGHT: Achieve lean!
DAY SIX: _____

WEEK EIGHT INTENTION (Repeat aloud 5 times in the morning and 5 times at night. Repeat silently 3 times prior to each meal):

I AM STRONG AND LEAN

# Meal #1 (within one hour of awakening) Time: _____
Water = 16 oz. (must be completely consumed prior to eating)
Protein = ___ g: _____
Fruit = small to medium piece
Carbohydrate = 1 cup non-instant oatmeal OR slice whole grain bread
Vegetable = 2 T flax, wheat germ, dried greens
Fish Oil capsules = 2 @ 300 mg total combined EPA & DHA (from sardines, anchovies, salmon, mackerel)

# Meal #2 (3 hours later) Time: _____
Water = 16 oz. (must be completely consumed prior to eating)
Protein = ___ g: _____
Vegetable = 1 serving fresh or frozen – lightly steamed, roasted or baked

# Meal #3 (3 hours later) Time: _____
Water = 16 oz. (must be completely consumed prior to eating)
Protein = ___ g: _____
Vegetable = 1-2 servings fresh or frozen – lightly steamed, roasted or baked
Fish Oil capsules = 2 @ 300 mg total combined EPA & DHA (from sardines, anchovies, salmon, mackerel)

Meal #4 (3 hours later) Time: _____
Water = 16 oz. (must be completely consumed prior to eating)
Protein = ___ g: _____
Nuts = ¼ cup OR Vegetable = 1 serving fresh or frozen – lightly steamed, roasted or baked

Meal #5 (3 hours later) Time: _____
Water = 16 oz. (must be completely consumed prior to eating)
Protein = ___ g: _____
Vegetable = 2-3 servings fresh or frozen – lightly steamed, roasted or baked
NO additional foods consumed

WEEK EIGHT: Achieve lean!
DAY SEVEN: _____

WEEK EIGHT INTENTION (Repeat aloud 5 times in the morning and 5 times at night. Repeat silently 3 times prior to each meal):

I AM STRONG AND LEAN

Meal #1 (within one hour of awakening) Time: _____
Water = 16 oz. (must be completely consumed prior to eating)
Protein = ___ g: _____
Fruit = small to medium piece
Carbohydrate = 1 cup non-instant oatmeal OR slice whole grain bread
Vegetable = 2 T flax, wheat germ, dried greens
Fish Oil capsules = 2 @ 300 mg total combined EPA & DHA (from sardines, anchovies, salmon, mackerel)

Meal #2 (3 hours later) Time: _____
Water = 16 oz. (must be completely consumed prior to eating)
Protein = ___ g: _____
Vegetable = 1 serving fresh or frozen – lightly steamed, roasted or baked

Meal #3 (3 hours later) Time: _____
Water = 16 oz. (must be completely consumed prior to eating)
Protein = ___ g: _____
Vegetable = 1-2 servings fresh or frozen – lightly steamed, roasted or baked
Fish Oil capsules = 2 @ 300 mg total combined EPA & DHA (from sardines, anchovies, salmon, mackerel)

Meal #4 (3 hours later) Time: _____

Water = 16 oz. (must be completely consumed prior to eating)

Protein = ___ g: _____

Nuts = ¼ cup OR Vegetable = 1 serving fresh or frozen – lightly steamed, roasted or baked

Meal #5 (3 hours later) Time: _____

Water = 16 oz. (must be completely consumed prior to eating)

Protein = ___ g: _____

Vegetable = 2-3 servings fresh or frozen – lightly steamed, roasted or baked

NO additional foods consumed